THE CURRENT STATUS AND FUTURE
OF ACADEMIC PEDIATRICS

Edited by
Elizabeth F. Purcell

THE CURRENT STATUS AND FUTURE
OF ACADEMIC PEDIATRICS

Report of a Conference
Sponsored Jointly by the
National Institute of Child
Health and Human Development
and the
Josiah Macy, Jr. Foundation

JOSIAH MACY, JR. FOUNDATION
One Rockeller Plaza, New York, New York 10020

© 1981 Josiah Macy, Jr. Foundation

All rights reserved

LIBRARY OF CONGRESS CATALOG CARD No.: 81-80922

    Purcell, Elizabeth F.

    The Current Status and Future of Academic Pediatrics
New York: Josiah Macy, Jr. Foundation, The

    240 pp.

    8104   810309

ISBN: 0-914362-36-4

Manufactured by the Heffernan Press, Worcester, Massachusetts

Distributed by the Independent Publishers Group

14 Vanderventer Avenue, Port Washington, New York 11050

CONTENTS

Discussant:
Henry L. Barnett 221
How Do We Meet the Needs?
William G. Anylan 226

PREFACE

This book is a companion to the volume entitled *The Current Status and Future of Academic Obstetrics* published in 1980 by the Josiah Macy, Jr. Foundation with the cooperation of the National Institute of Child Health and Human Development (NICHD). This book, like the previous one, derives from a conference, this time held in New Orleans on 22 to 24 June 1980.

The Macy Foundation and the NICHD have a continuing interest in fostering the scientific and educational aspirations of academic pediatrics and academic obstetrics because these are the fields of medicine most concerned with human development. Together, then, these two volumes present a current assessment of the two disciplines, their histories, constructs, and needs.

Pediatrics has evolved as a distinct branch of medicine only since the nineteenth century. Until the turn of this century no single medical specialty had focused specifically on the child. In the early 1900s the field concentrated primarily on the scourges afflicting children and on general aspects of child health and development. It was not until 1903, however, that Harvard Medical School appointed Thomas Morgan Rotch as the first true professor of pediatrics in this country.

In the past two decades pediatrics has gained momentum as a scientific discipline and medical specialty responsive to the needs of children. For example, pediatrics was in the forefront of the child welfare movement and of research on diarrhea, nutrition, infection, human genetics, and development; more recently it has played a large role in the emerging emphasis on the behavioral sciences and ambulatory medicine. Within that perspective the participants in this conference agreed that three factors would continue to have a great effect on the future of academic pediatrics.

One of these is the unrelenting trend toward subspecialization—particularly neonatology, allergy, and cardiology. A second major consideration is that academic pediatrics is facing a future beset by a decrease in federal support for research and training. The third trend is a heavier reliance on funds from clinical services necessitated by the decline of federal sources; this means faculty pediatricians will have less time available for teaching and research in a field already troubled by a shortage of clinical investigators.

As mentioned earlier, pediatrics has always been responsive to social currents, but it is now incumbent on the leaders of academic pediatrics to examine and reflect on their discipline and the political, social, and economic factors that affect it, as well as to work to shape the pediatrics of tomorrow.

It would be inappropriate for me to conclude this preface without acknowledging our deep indebtedness to John Z. Bowers, M.D., who retired as president of the Macy Foundation in September 1980. In working together to plan this conference and the earlier one on academic obstetrics, Dr. Bowers's advice and counsel was always provocative and on target. On behalf of the NICHD I should like to express our gratitude to John Bowers and the Macy Foundation for their willing cooperation in these two ventures.

Norman Kretchmer, M.D., Ph.D.
Director
National Institute of Child Health
and Human Development

THE EVOLUTION OF ACADEMIC PEDIATRICS IN THE PAST TWENTY-FIVE YEARS

Horace L. Hodes

One of the meanings of "evolution," the operative word in the title of the subject assigned to me, is "the process of developing from a rudimentary to a complete state." I do not believe that academic pediatrics has reached a complete and final state, but it is true that experiences over the past twenty-five years have had a maturing influence. During that period academic pediatrics has undergone an extreme expansion in size and complexity in its biomedical and psychosocial activities. Nothing that involves children, their families, their environment, and their community is outside the present-day domain of academic pediatrics.

The technological advances that have improved the chance for survival of the premature or of the infant with some form of serious congenital defect have involved us much more heavily in neonatology than was the case twenty-five years ago. Moreover, in most academic centers pediatrics has assumed the responsibility for adolescent medicine. This development has opened new areas for research in such fields as nutrition and endocrinology, and has brought us face-to-face with social, psychosexual, and family problems that makes life in departments of pediatrics quite hectic at times.

Academic pediatrics is no longer "academic" in the ivory tower sense. We are deeply involved with the lives of our patients and our communities. Furthermore we are constantly reminded that the actions of local, state, and federal governments directly affect our daily work and our professional and intellectual endeavors to a much greater extent than they did in 1955.

I am sure the academic pediatric community will agree, however, that not all of the maturation process has been pleasant or productive; and, since the process is continuing, at least minor readjustments are in store for us. While my personal estimation of the changes that have occurred is on the whole very positive, some developments, which I shall touch on later, do not seem to be in the best interests of children or of pediatrics.

In the past quarter-century the number of academic pediatric departments in the United States expanded materially due to the transformation of nonacademic departments into academic ones and to the formation of new medical schools that began with academic departments of pediatrics. In addition, over the same period the number of pediatric faculty members increased at a rate that was not conceived of in the preceding decade.

EXPANSION OF RESEARCH

There are a number of reasons for these developments. The 1950s saw a growing acceptance of the value of research on the part of the American public and government. The belief that the most difficult health problems could be solved by research became widespread, and financial support for biomedical science was raised to a level not previously available. The signing in 1950 of the Omnibus Medical Research Act authorized the creation of the National Institutes of Health (NIH). Of great significance to pediatrics was the establishment in 1963 of the National Institute of Child Health and Human Development (NICHD); also important to academic pediatrics was the founding of the Institute of General Medical Sciences in the same year.

Norman Kretchmer will probably speak at greater length about the influence of the NICHD on research and academic training in departments of pediatrics. I shall merely say that the growth and achievements of academic pediatrics since 1963 would not have been possible without the support of the NICHD. The role of the NIH in the development of academic pediatrics is indicated by the financial support it has given over the years to departments of pediatrics and to children's hospitals: from 1968 through 1979 the NICHD and certain other NIH agencies granted to such institutions a total of $800 million, ranging from a low of $40 million in 1970 to a high of $108 million in 1979; the average annual sum awarded by the NIH has been close to $67 million. Even allowing for inflation these are very impressive figures.

The amount of money awarded for research depends not only on the merit of the research proposal but on public opinion and pressure and on the wishes of the Congress. Thus research on cancer, heart disease, stroke, neurological diseases, and blindness are specifically mandated by acts of Congress. At least one public law mandates that the NICHD carry out specific studies. Public Law 93-270, enacted on 22 April 1974, for example, directed the secretary of the Department of Health, Education, and Welfare (DHEW), through the agency of the NICHD, to carry out specific and general research on the sudden infant death syndrome and to submit a report on this subject to the Congress.

Not only has academic pediatrics grown in size and complexity, it has grown and changed in another way. The number of departments influential in research, training, and innovative clinical pediatrics has multiplied, and such departments are now found in all parts of the country. In 1955 a few leading centers were scattered in the South and on the West Coast, but leadership in pediatrics was primarily in centers in the Northeast and the Midwest; a much more even national distribution exists today, with the Southwest and West well represented by outstanding pediatric departments.

ADEQUACY OF TRAINING

In the late 1950s leaders of academic pediatrics became aware that many pediatricians they had trained felt inadequately prepared to deal with the patients they encountered daily in their practice. This feeling was clearly documented in a survey conducted in 1958 by Robert A. Aldrich, who asked: "How does your practice differ from what you had anticipated when entering pediatrics?" The question was addressed to 2,000 pediatricians across the country, and 1,164 replied. Fewer than 36 percent, most of whom were in the older age group, reported "no significant difference" between what they had expected and what they actually found; the remaining 64 percent said they had faced unanticipated problems. It is interesting—but not of direct relevance to our subject—that 20 percent found working hours excessive, and that 21 percent complained of lack of professional status, unnecessary telephone calls, and inconsiderate, demanding parents. It is of significance that 36 percent stated they had to deal with a great many more well patients than anticipated, and 11 percent found an unexpectedly high ratio of emotional and behavioral problems among their patients. Aldrich's survey showed that in 1958 a typical pediatrician's day was spent in caring for patients in the following categories: well-child care and emotional and behavioral problems, 35 percent; respiratory infections, 28 percent; gastrointestinal disturbances, 10 percent; allergies, 8 percent; accidents, 6 percent; and all others, 13 percent.

PRESCRIPTION FOR CHANGE

Quite apart from the impetus provided by the complaints of practicing pediatricians, everyone working in academic pediatrics recognized that changes had to be made in the direction of pediatric training. The title of Samuel Levine's presidential address to the American Pediatric Society in 1969 was "Pediatric Education at the Cross Roads." In it he outlined the changes and additions he believed should be made in the pediatric curriculum, from the first year of medical school through the final year of residency. It is quite remarkable to see how closely most departments of academic pediatrics today conform to the pattern Levine recommended: one cannot escape the belief that his proposals had a tremendous influence on the direction taken by pediatrics. For this reason I will quote a slightly edited version of his prescription:

• Increased emphasis on human embryology, with special reference to prematurity, genetic diseases, and congenital malformations.

• More attention to infant and child growth and development, including mental, emotional, and social, as well as physical, characteristics.

• Greater and more imaginative use of outpatient services, including the emergency unit and the follow-up, well-baby, toddler, and school-age clinics.

• Closer contact with prospective parents; experience in premature and newborn nurseries; and emphasis on home visits during the postnatal period and later.

• More continuous collaboration with psychologists, psychiatrists, and sociologists, particularly concerning behavioral problems, Greater familiarity with official and voluntary agencies devoted to child health and welfare.

• A special effort to understand the problems and potentials of adolescents.

• More frequent contact, as a medical student and as a resident, with both normal children and normal parents.

• More day-to-day dealings with mentally retarded, physically handicapped, and emotionally disturbed children.

• A brighter focus on the world of the schoolroom, particularly on problems of vision, hearing, speech, and reading.

Levine concluded his landmark paper by saying that "the young pediatrician today . . . faces a real opportunity to promote all aspects of child life and health in his community—mental, moral, emotional, and social, as well as just physical."

The implication of this statement was that academic pediatrics must expand its mission to include some neglected biomedical aspects of child health, and that it must include psychosocial considerations within its discipline. In no way, however, did he convey the idea that pediatrics should depart from the most rigorous standards of biomedical research.

CONTACT WITH PARENTS

It is of interest that Levine's recommendation that pediatricians in training should have closer contact with parents has come about in the hospital despite the objections of administrators, departments of nursing, and some pediatricians. In the 1950s even "progressive" hospitals and clinics severely limited parents' visits to their children. With the introduction of effective antibiotics the need for such a restriction disappeared, but it was continued in some hospitals because it was convenient for the staff. Eventually, under pressure, the restriction was removed, and in most children's services today visits by parents are normal features of the daily hospital routine. In fact many parents spend the day with their children, and some stay overnight at the hospital. Hospitals now encourage this practice and make housekeeping arrangements that facilitate it. This development has of course been of great benefit to hospitalized children, as well as a comfort to the parents.

The constant presence of parents in the hospital setting has also had extremely beneficial effects on pediatricians. Students and house officers learn from the very beginning that every measure they take or plan to take must take into account the reaction of a child's parents. Furthermore they must explain the logic of their thinking and planning to the parents, and make clear the value and need for any procedure under consideration. This is especially true if it causes inconvenience or distress or pain to the child.

House officers trained in the modern pediatric clinic deal constantly with complicated socioeconomic problems and realize that they are an integral part of the profession. They know they will deal with them in the practice of pediatrics, whether in a full-time academic setting or in a group or solo practice. Pediatricians who complete their formal training today are very much better prepared than were their predecessors of the 1950s or 1960s. I have no statistics on this point, but I believe the pediatricians who were trained in the 1970s and who are now in practice are a happier and more contented lot than those who preceded them.

It occurs to me that the constant presence of parents on hospital wards may have an effect on the career selection of our medical students. Those who feel they would not be willing to deal with the complex relationship of physician and patient, together with the family, might very well decide against pediatrics as a profession. I do not suggest this is the only reason that a student might choose another field of medicine as a career, but it may have some influence.

RECRUITMENT OF PEDIATRICIANS

This may be a good point to make some general observations about the recruitment of physicians to pediatrics. It is natural for practicing and academic pediatricians to be concerned about the number and quality of the physicians entering their branch of medicine. This concern has probably been intensified because of the particular stresses that have been placed on pediatrics. Anyone who has frequent contact with medical students is called on to give advice about their postgraduate training and their career options. Those of us who teach pediatrics are frequently requested to help students choose between pediatrics and other medical disciplines. These students have already narrowed their choice to a medical, as opposed to a surgical, subspecialty career, and they have almost always eliminated psychiatry as a possibility. In my own experience the student has very often come close to a decision before our discussion begins. This is not always the case, however, and in these instances the advisor often learns what the factors are that persuade a student not to choose pediatrics.

I shall summarize the antipediatric influences as I understand them from my own experience; they are very similar to the findings of two women pediatricians who are associate deans for third- and fourth-year medical students.

It is true that the factors cited by students may not correspond to reality, but they are the students' concepts of the situation that exists in pediatrics. Some give economic reasons, expressing the fear that the declining birth rate may make it difficult for new practitioners to establish themselves. Some see themselves in competition with nurse practitioners and with physicians trained in family medicine. One frequent complaint is that a great deal of the pediatrician's time is taken up with such minor matters as well-baby care, routine immunizations, and other services that can be provided by those with less rigorous training, and that, in any event, such work is neither interesting nor challenging. On occasion a student will say that she/he finds pediatrics at least as appealing as medicine, if not more so, but that internal medicine will be the choice because the income to be earned in that specialty is so much greater.

It is quite clear that the competition for a general medical residency is much more severe than it is for pediatric house staff positions; an analysis of the results of the 1980 National Internship and Residency Matching Program confirms this fact. A statistically significantly larger percentage of pediatric internships remain unfilled than is the case for positions in internal medicine. The causes of this are not clear, but they are probably multiple. Of the 1,802 internships in pediatrics offered, 1,318 (73 percent) were filled; 484 (27 percent) were not filled. This is almost exactly the same as the failure rate for internships and residencies in all categories: 4,400 (25 percent) of the 18,000 positions available remained unfilled. In contrast to the results obtained in the "all categories" group and in pediatrics only, 842 (17 percent) of the 4,891 positions offered in internal medicine were not filled. Statistical comparison of the results in medicine and pediatrics gives a chi-square value of 77 (p is less than 0.0001).

WOMEN IN MEDICINE

Until recently a much higher percentage of American women graduates went into pediatrics than into internal medicine. This was partly due to their preference and partly because their acceptance as residents in internal medicine was not as wholehearted as it was in pediatrics. In 1955—the beginning of the quarter-century under discussion—about 6 percent of medical school applicants were women, and they made up about 6 percent of each entering class. During the 1960s there was a gradual rise in the percentage of women candidates applying for admission to medical school, and a corresponding increase in their acceptance. Beginning in 1970 a very sharp rise occurred in the number of women applicants, and a concomitant rise in the number accepted. In 1980–81 almost 30 percent of the applicants, and 28.9 percent of those accepted to American medical schools, are women.

Arnold S. Relman described these developments in some detail in a recent editorial in the *New England Journal of Medicine*. He stated that pediatrics is no longer the favored career choice of women medical graduates, and that: "Internal medicine, virtually shunned in the past, is now the favored specialty among women graduates."[1] Relman mentioned, also, that family practice has been attracting an increasing number of women; this discipline is probably attracting an appreciable percentage of men and women who in previous years might have chosen pediatrics.

CONTRIBUTIONS TO RESEARCH

Other participants in this conference will describe the impacts of endocrinology, neurobiology, genetics, perinatology, nutrition, and behavioral sciences on the development of pediatrics. Faculty members of the department of pediatrics have of course contributed very materially to these sciences. Most of the studies in genetics conducted in American schools, for example, are carried out in departments of pediatrics rather than in internal medicine or obstetrics. Similarly, in most institutions prenatal diagnosis and genetic counseling are conducted in departments of pediatrics. It is certainly clear that pediatricians have contributed a great deal to research in genetics and have been the leaders in research on chromosome banding and subbanding and on chromatid damage.

Microbiology

Since no other speaker has been assigned to the topic of the impact of microbiology on pediatrics, I shall speak to that point. In the late 1950s many people believed that the most fruitful research in microbiology had been completed, and students were advised to work in other medical sciences. This opinion proved to be completely incorrect, and pediatricians have played a very important part in the spectacular discoveries in microbiology during the last twenty years; academic pediatrics made essential contributions to the scientific advances in microbiology and infectious diseases, and pediatricians were largely responsible for the work that led to the discovery and development of vaccines for poliomyelitis, measles, mumps, and rubella.

Pediatricians were also the major contributors to advances in our knowledge of intrauterine and congenital infections such as toxoplasmosis rubella, cytomegalovirus disease, and herpes. Their recent work includes the demonstration of the late effects of these infections on hearing, vision, and mental development. This is a valuable contribution to the understanding of the factors that may be involved in developmental disorders.

The work of pediatricians on the virology and epidemiology of respiratory viruses such as a parainfluenza, adenoviruses, and R-S virus has demonstrated the significance of respiratory viral disease in early life; by using parainfluenza virus as a model they discovered some of the important mechanisms in the production of persistent viral infections.

Pediatricians have made many very interesting discoveries about the etiology and pathogenesis of infectious gastroenteritis. These include the discovery of plasmid-induced toxins of *E. coli,* which are responsible for a great deal of bacterial gastroenteritis found everywhere in the world. The same can be said about the discovery of the colonization factor plasmids that enable these organisms to adhere to the mucosa of the intestine and thereby permit their toxins to cause gastroenteritis. Pediatricians played a key role in the discovery of the importance of Campylobacter and Yersinia as etiological agents of infantile diarrhea, and they described infant botulism and chlamydial disease of early infancy.

American, Australian, and English pediatricians did most of the work in the discovery of the diarrhea viruses and clarified their epidemiology. They isolated and cultured the rotaviruses, and showed that they are the most common cause of diarrhea in children under age five. They were instrumental also in the discovery of the parvovirus, astrovirus, and calicivirus gastroenteritis. Pediatricians are actively engaged in research with antiviral agents such as adenine arabinoside and acyclo guanosine. Some members of pediatric departments are working in the very interesting subspecialty of recombinant DNA research. One such group has very recently combined the genome of type B hepatitis virus with an *E. coli* plasmid that mediates penicillinase production by the bacterium. After the combined plasmid was manufactured in great quantities by the *E. coli* the viral genome was removed by restriction enzymes; it was then recirculated and made to enter HeLa cells growing in tissue culture. These cells, which are of human origin, multiplied and produced the surface antigen of hepatitis B antigen and secreted it into the medium.

Virtually every academic department of pediatrics is involved in research in the behavioral sciences and in studies dealing with the provision of medical care. I do not know exactly how much of the funds spent on research in pediatrics is devoted to work in these categories—Kretchmer may speak to that point. I do know that 45 percent of the extramural grants awarded by the NICHD in 1970 was for behavioral research. Gerald D. LaVeck, then director of the NICHD, stated that such a large proportion of research money was awarded to psychology projects because the grading of applications by the psychology study sections was much more lenient than that of their counterparts in biology and medicine. At present the NICHD awards only 20 to 25 percent of its extramural funds to behavioral sciences. A number of academic pediatricians believe this trend should be accelerated because of the conviction that psychosocial research in pediatrics has on the whole been unproductive.

The last point I shall make is that the kind of patient treated in pediatric services has changed. The number of children with infections has decreased, but those with chronic illness, congenital disease, and illnesses common to adolescents have increased. One children's hospital recently reported that 50 percent of its inpatients suffered from a familial disease caused by a single gene defect or from a developmental deficiency. In our own hospital, 22 percent of the pediatric department inpatients are adolescents.

NOTE

1. Arnold S. Relman, "Here Come the Women," *New England Journal of Medicine* 302 (1980): 1252–53.

DISCUSSANT

Margaret H. D. Smith

Several striking changes have occurred in academic pediatrics in the last forty years. Basic is the fact that pediatrics is now a required subject in the curricula of all American medical schools. This was not always so. Prior to the 1940s in many medical schools it was an elective, albeit a popular one.

A second significant development is the change in the diseases with which pediatrics is now primarily concerned— what Robert J. Haggerty has called "the new morbidity"[1]—such as the behavioral and social disturbances and adolescent problems that are currently taking precedence over the nutritional and infectious disease problem of the very young that were formerly the main province of pediatrics. In the early 1940s, for example, only children up to age four years were admitted to the Pediatric Service at Charity Hospital in New Orleans; children over that age were attended by internists.

Another great change in pediatrics has been the proliferation of subspecialties. Formerly the well-rounded pediatrician was expected to have mastered the discipline completely, and it was in fact possible to do so; now the body of knowledge is too vast to encompass. Subspecialization is important, also, because it promotes basic research, and academic careers are predicated on research, and on the publications engendered therefrom. In the area of clinical investigation, subspecialization is as crucial to pediatrics as it is to adult medicine because it attracts patients in greater numbers to the academic medical center, thereby contributing to the financial support of the faculty.

There are, however, drawbacks to subspecialization. The

discipline encompasses all the medical problems of the young, growing individual. It therefore includes both general medicine applied to this age group as well as all the special medical problems. But inevitable fragmentation of teaching makes it difficult for house officers and medical students to gain a reasonable perspective of the field. It also creates administrative and personal problems in large group practices, both academic and nonacademic, because, for example, the subspecialists need more time for each appointment and therefore charge higher fees than the "generalists".

One last striking change I wish to mention is travel, not only travel by the faculty, which has been much discussed and is in no way special to pediatrics, but the diminished mobility of house officers in training. Years ago it was customary for a student to go away to college, very likely to a private college that drew students from all over the country, and then on to medical school, again perhaps in another state. Next came the pediatric residency years when house officers usually moved to another location at least once, perhaps twice. Now it is more customary for a young person to attend a state college in or near home, a state medical school that admits only residents of that state, and then take a three-year residency in the same community. The mobility of former days ensured contact with leading professors of the day, exposure to a variety of medical and social problems, as well as contact with people with different laboratory and clinical interests and degrees of competence. In short it expanded the horizons of the pediatrician-in-training. I believe such broadening influences are of paramount importance in stimulating the inquiring mind and in helping patients and their families to maintain health in our mercurial society.

There is allegedly a crisis in academic psychiatry, academic obstetrics, and academic pediatrics. Why in these three specialities? What have they in common? I submit that they have in common the fact that all deal with the most mobile, most fragile members of our multiethnic, multiracial, multieverything, rapidly expanding society. Psychiatrists work with people either unable to adapt to the world as they find it, or who, having adapted, have broken down under stress. Obstetricians deal largely with young women and young couples under multiple psychological, social, and moral pressures. Pediatricians treat children and adolescents and their families who are changing incessantly in a changing world. In each case of course the problems are further compounded by the fact that as academics we are not usually observing the problems directly but are trying to teach medical students to develop a sensitive, inquiring, flexible attitude when confronting problems, both biological and social, and to seek satisfactory solutions. I believe the former custom of exposing house officers to two or three academic environments during their formative professional years contributed significantly to the development of imaginative, thoughtful, creative powers on the part of those going into academic careers. I would like to see a return to that kind of mobility.

NOTE

1. R. J. Haggerty, K. J. Roghmann, and I. B. Pless, *Child Health and the Community* (New York: John Wiley & Sons, 1975).

SUPPORT OF ACADEMIC PEDIATRICS

CURRENT PERSPECTIVES IN AND FEDERAL SUPPORT OF ACADEMIC PEDIATRICS

Norman Kretchmer

INTRODUCTION

The first department of pediatrics was established at the Karolinska Institute in Sweden in 1845. Academic pediatrics in America has had an interesting but relatively short history, however, having been introduced only 100 years ago.[1] It was not until late in the nineteenth century that pediatrics separated from internal medicine as a distinct branch of medicine with a unique focus—the child. By 1900 a dozen children's hospitals had been established, and sixty-four special chairs of pediatrics had been endowed in 119 medical schools. Thomas Morgan Rotch, appointed to a chair on the Harvard Medical School faculty in 1903, was the first true professor of pediatrics in the United States.

That was the era of the giants and the founders of the field of pediatrics. Abraham Jacobi, who came to this country from his native Germany in 1853, established the field of pediatrics, adamantly stating that infants and children were unique and could not be thought of or treated as young adults. He was clinical professor of diseases of children at Babies Hospital, New York Medical College, and his writings in the field are classics; Job Lewis Smith was a socially conscious pediatrician concerned about housing and disease in the shantytown located in the area of Central Park in New York; Emmet Holt, Sr. succeeded Jacobi at Babies Hospital, where he set up a research laboratory; John Howland, another who would influence the field, organized the second pediatric research laboratory at Baltimore's Harriet Lane Home in 1912. Both Holt and Howland integrated their clinical work with basic science activities.

These four men put down the roots of modern American pediatrics, and their concerns are reflected in our present-day activities. Each helped to establish the emphasis of pediatrics today: social welfare; the child in society; human development; clinical medicine and teaching; and basic research.

It was Holt who in 1923, during his second tenure as president of the American Pediatric Society predicted that in the years to come three distinct types of pediatricians would emerge—first, the researcher, who would probably be a full-time head of a department of pediatrics in a university medical school; second, the individual who would apply our best science in the treatment of sick children; and third, the public health pediatricians.

According to Holt it was important to predict who among these would be the most essential. Emphasizing teaching as a primary task of the physician, and especially of the pediatrician of the future, he went on to say that comparatively few at that time had the training, the opportunity, or the resources for profitable scientific research. Every day it was becoming more difficult to be properly fitted for such work. . . . "But all of us can have a share and a large one, in this general campaign of education which must form the basis of great achievements in the field of preventive medicine."[2] Pediatrics has continued along the path of Holt's prophecy.

Another element that was to enter the field of medicine was specialization—as predicted by another president of the American Pediatric Society, William Osler, who in 1892 said: "The rapid increase in knowledge has made concentration in work a necessity. Specialism is here and here to stay. Let the younger of my hearers take this to heart. . . ."[3]

These statements by the earlier pediatricians serve as a basis for the discussion to follow. But, in my view, there is another force that has guided and continues to influence the specialty—pediatrics has been the medical field most responsive to the current needs of society. Take, for examples, the child welfare movement; the extensive research on diarrhea, electrolytes, nutrition, infection, human genetics, and development; and more recently the emphasis on the behavioral sciences and ambulatory medicine. The development of academic pediatrics over the past decades has been dictated by the needs of society, tempered by the availability of funds as well as by the particular schools of thought that have emerged in the discipline. The funds needed to gain a foothold have derived mainly from federal sources, particularly from the National Institutes of Health (NIH), reaching a zenith in the 1960s; this financial stimulus to growth persisted up to the early 1970s, and then began to wane.

A number of concerns occupied the heads of pediatrics departments, including:
- The development of subspecialties.
- The recruitment of faculty.
- The acquisition of space and money for research.
- The availability of clinical facilities for undergraduate and postgraduate teaching.
- The gathering of a cadre of young people, derived locally or from other institutions, who wanted to pursue careers in academic medicine.

In the 1950s it became apparent that in order to establish a career in academic pediatrics an individual had to obtain subspecialty training *and* a capability for research in a specific area, either following or in concert with clinical training. The ability to accomplish this objective was possible in the 1950s and 1960s, improbable in the 1970s, and almost impossible in the 1980s.

Concurrent with the availability of increased funds from the NIH, and particularly with the establishment of the National Institute of Child Health and Human Development (NICHD) in 1963, a striking change began to occur in American pediatrics. Over the past two decades the proportion of graduates selecting pediatrics as a specialty has increased from 6 to 10 percent. This trend is in part due to the heightened emphasis on primary care, that is, on pediatrics, internal medicine, and family practice. Among the specialties, pediatrics today maintains a position of fourth in popularity, preceded by internal medicine, surgery, and family practice, in that order.

Within academic departments of pediatrics there has been an upsurge of interest in subspecialization. This trend is clearly demonstrated by the subspecialties in the Department of Pediatrics at Cornell University–New York Hospital Medical Center between 1960 and 1980 (Table 1),* and in the Department of Pediatrics of the University of California–San Francisco Medical Center (UCSF) from 1970 to 1980 (Table 2). It is interesting that adolescent medicine had disappeared as a speciality at Cornell by 1965, but was reestablished in 1974. Ambulatory care, mental health, and oncology also became fields of special interest in the 1970s. At UCSF there were similar

TABLE 1. CORNELL UNIVERSITY–NEW YORK HOSPITAL MEDICAL CENTER,
SPECIALTIES WITHIN THE DEPARTMENT OF PEDIATRICS, 1960,
AND OTHER SPECIALTIES ADDED BY 1980[1]

1960	Added by 1980
Adolescent Clinic[2]	Allergy and Immunology
Allergy Clinic	Ambulatory Care
Cardiology	Dermatology
Endocrinology and	Diabetes Clinic[4]
Metabolic Diseases	Hematology/Oncology
Gastroenterology Clinic[3]	High-Risk Follow-Up Clinic
General Pediatric Clinic	Hypertension Clinic
Hematology	Infectious Diseases
Transfusion Clinic	Mental Health
Premature Follow-Up Clinic	Neonatology
Renal Clinic	Neurology
Rheumatic Fever Clinic	Pediatric Nephrology
	Transplantation and Dialysis
	Follow-Up Clinic
	Rheumatic Diseases
	Surgical Follow-Up Clinic
	Pediatric Urology

NOTES: 1) Wallace McCrory, chairman, Department of Pediatrics, 1961–80: personal communication. 2) Discontinued in 1965; reestablished in 1974. 3) Discontinued in 1978. 4) Within endocrinology and metabolic diseases.

---

* The data for departments of pediatrics and children's hospital shown in Tables 1 through 7 represent only a portion of the total support of these sources by the National Institutes of Health and the National Institute of Child Health and Human Development. The data were retrieved by means of a computer system that stores information taken directly from research grant applications. If the investigator is a faculty member in pediatrics but failed to indicate that fact, the department is not credited with the research. The figures shown therefore represent a minimum level of support.

TABLE 2. UNIVERSITY OF CALIFORNIA–SAN FRANCISCO MEDICAL CENTER,
SPECIALTIES WITHIN THE DEPARTMENT OF PEDIATRICS, 1970,
AND OTHER SPECIALTIES ADDED BY 1980

1970	Added by 1980
Allergy	Ambulatory and Community
Behavioral Pediatrics	Pediatrics
Cardiology	Adolescent Medicine
Endocrinology	Clinical Pharmacology
Infectious Diseases	Gastroenterology
Neonatology	Genetics
	Hematology/Oncology
	Intensive Care Pediatrics
	Nephrology and Nutrition
	Neurology
	Pulmonary Diseases

changes, with the addition by 1980 of clinical pharmacology and intensive care pediatrics.

The position of this subspecialty in academic medicine was further strengthened by the development of subspecialty boards in its various fields; 56 percent of pediatricians entering subspecialties today favor four areas: neonatology (23 percent); allergy (15 percent): behavior (10 percent); and adolescence (8 percent).

This major trend toward subspecialization has resulted in intellectual fragmentation of departments of pediatrics, and as a consequence they bear less of a resemblance to cohesive units and more to conglomerates of separate hefdoms. Specialization is important, perhaps imperative, in the face of the vast store of knowledge being accumulated; at the same time, however, the amalgamating force in a department should focus on the child and the concept of human development, which can serve as the medium to hold a department together in the atmosphere of present stresses.

In the past decade there has been pressure, mainly from the American public as represented by both houses of Congress, to drastically expand the country's medical force. In fact in 1976 Surgeon General W.H. Steward, himself a pediatrician, went on record as predicting that by 1980 we would require nearly 75,000 pediatricians.[4] The number of medical schools increased from eighty-four in 1970 to 125 in 1980, fostered and abetted by the lure of student capitation monies. What dean or legislator could resist so overt a temptation? Today capitation money is being discontinued, and the country is left with an overwhelming, expensive national medical structure.

These financial incentives of the past led to enormous increases in clinical faculty—from 7,300 in 1960, to 19,000 in 1970, to 33,000 in 1977. Overall there was an expansion of pediatric faculty from 1,500 in 1967 to 3,500 in 1977.[5] Simplistically, the ability of medical schools to expand was enhanced by the influx of large amounts of funds from the NIH; capitation funds from the Health Resources Administration (HRA); and third-party payments from public sources.

The financial wellspring has dried up in the past decade because of curtailment of the federal budget and because inflationary trends have caused the dollar to lose half its purchasing power. The result has been the emergence of two phenomena: first, an attempt by academic medical centers to continue the growth of the past, or at least to maintain an affluent status quo; and, second, the acquisition and utilization of more and more money derived from direct service activities. From 1964 to 1974 federal funds in support of academic medical centers increased in actual dollars from $268 million to $493 million; but the *percentage* of funds from federal sources dropped from 36 to 21, while funds from local and state sources rose from 13 to 20 percent, and income from professional fees rose from 4 to 22 percent.

This mix of sources of support is not a transient occurrence; it is likely to prevail and intensify if it is not actively controlled. The penchant for preserving the status quo and the reliance on funds from the provision of services are truly threatening, for there is no way that academic medicine can continue its disorganized, unplanned growth. The use of service activities as a major fiscal source can only lead to infringement on the time necessary for other academic pursuits. These developments are usually least effective in a department of pediatrics, for the pediatrician, whether a subspecialist or generalist, is invariably the lowest income producer in the medical community, Thus reliance on service earnings is not only a danger to academic medicine, but often futile in academic pediatrics.

Federal Support for Departments of Pediatrics

In order to understand the impact of federal support on departments of pediatrics it is helpful to have a general idea of the broader budgetary and historic context in which it occurred. In 1976 the President's Biomedical Research Panel published a study of the effects of federal funds, particularly health research funds, on academic medical centers.[6] I would like to review some of the conclusions and impressions of the panel, for I believe they still hold today even though the study covered data available only up to 1974. Current fiscal trends have heightened the impact of the findings of the panel, and I have updated its data with figures from the NIH and the Association of American Medical Colleges (AAMC).

FINANCIAL LINKS BETWEEN THE FEDERAL GOVERNMENT AND ACADEMIA

An adequate health research effort requires a network of financially sound and educationally viable academic institutions. It was clear to the panel, as it is to all involved in academic medicine, that the federal government and academic medical centers are bound together inextricably as a result of the rapid growth of federal support for biomedical research that began in the early 1950s. Medical schools have developed programs counting on an inflow of federal monies, particularly for research, and government programs have evolved with the understanding that academic institutions will conduct most of the research.

It is estimated that in fiscal year 1980 the federal government will support about 62 percent of health research in this country, with 42 percent coming from the NIH (Figure 1);[7] industry will support about 29 percent, mostly for *development* rather than health research; and other sources account for 9 percent. The total dollar amount is close to $8 billion. These percentages have held fairly constant since 1975, but the total dollar amount, calculated against 1969 constant dollars, is only $3.5 billion. Thus the real purchasing power is 50 percent of what it was in 1969.

Figure 2 shows who conducts the health research: of the

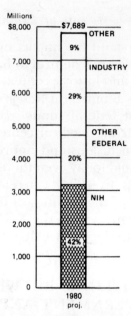

Figure 1. Support for health research in the United States, by source, 1980 (estimated).

Source: Department of Health and Human Services, *Basic Data Relating to the National Institutes of Health,* NIH publication no. 80-1261 (Bethesda: National Institutes of Health, 1980).

total estimated federal outflow in 1979, 51 percent went to institutions of higher education; NIH funds to these institutions were higher—60 percent. Very little money from industry went to academic institutions; 79 percent of its funds was spent intramurally.

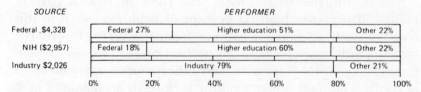

Figure 2. Support for health research in the United States, by source and performer, 1979 (estimated). In millions of dollars.

Source: Department of Health and Human Services, *Basic Data Relating to the National Institutes of Health,* NIH publication no. 80-1261 (Bethesda: National Institutes of Health, 1980).

Not all the money flowing to academic institutions is in the form of research funds. The federal government is involved in the support of all three major pursuits of academic institutions: research; education—mainly from the HRA for *capitation* and *residency training;* and patient care—mainly from the Health Services Administration (HSA) and from Medicaid/Medicare reimbursements through the Health Care Financing Administration. Nevertheless federal funds for research represent a large share of the total support given to academic institutions. According to figures released by the AAMC in 1977, the last year for which data were reported, 25 percent of medical school revenues came in the form of federal research funds; only about 7 percent came from other federal programs such as capitation and grants relating to patient service. The President's Biomedical Research Panel found that this research money has a profound effect on the organization and operation of these institutions.

Changing Trends in Federal Support for Academic Medicine

Academic medicine has expanded rapidly since World War II. In the late 1950s and early 1960s growth was stimulated by the expansion of biomedical research supported by the NIH: their funds to academic medical centers rose from $8.2 million in 1950 to $618 million in 1973. There was a concomitant expansion of graduate research training programs to provide basic and clinical scientists for this growing effort—from $4 million in 1950 to $170 million in 1970. By fiscal year 1979 the NIH had awarded over $1 billion to the medical schools for research and research training.

In about 1968 American medical centers experienced a spurt in growth. Medical schools increased student enrollments as the public exerted pressure for more physicians and the federal government offered incentives in the form of HRA capitation funds to expand class sizes. At the same time, the schools widened their commitments to train and educate other professionals and technical personnel. New schools and existing schools were awarded federal funds for construction, student loans, scholarships, and operating costs.

The symbiotic relationship between the federal government and academic medicine had reached its zenith by 1968. In that year over 50 percent of the total revenues of the medical schools derived from federal sources; they also received increased support for their education programs from state governments, as well as from tuition, endowments, and private sources.

Over the next several years came gradual changes, which in retrospect were dramatic. The medical schools began to increase their emphasis on medical services. By 1974, according to the President's Biomedical Research Panel, academic medical centers were in the final phases of their evolution from primarily undergraduate institutions to sophisticated providers of advanced medical care, a move that meant a higher proportion of their operating budgets derived from clinical activities. Federal funds, especially research funds, declined as a fraction of the total budget revenue, and a larger share was contributed by state and local governments. According to data from the AAMC, federal resources dropped from 45 percent of the total revenues of medical schools in 1970, to 37 percent in 1975, to 32 percent in 1977; concomitantly, funds from state and local governments varied from 23 percent, to 28 percent, to 27 percent in those same years. Revenues from medical services, tuition, and fees rose from 14 percent in 1970, to 19 percent in 1975, to 28 percent in 1977. And there is no indication that these ratios have changed radically in 1980.

In summary, the budgetary importance of research programs has declined compared to other activities of academic medical centers, not because of an absolute decrease in research activities, but because of other demands to which the centers have responded. Academic medical centers today derive more than one-fifth of their support from patient fees, that is, from funds generated by the clinical faculty.

Effects of Research Funding on Academic Medicine

In its study the President's Biomedical Research Panel found that research funding—and changes in that funding— has had profound effects on academic medicine.

Federal funds for research support and training in basic medical sciences have the strongest impact on enrollment levels and on the production of Ph.D.'s; the production of M.D.'s, however, seems most strongly associated with health manpower funding. Medical student enrollments grew from 32,400 in 1964, to 50,000 in 1974, to 60,456 in 1978, while the number of M.D.'s graduating annually rose from 7,400 in 1964, to 11,600 in 1974, to 15,123 in 1979. Research funding seemed to have a neutral effect on the size of education programs for graduate physicians.

Not surprisingly the president's panel found that the size of medical school faculties increased as education programs expanded. Faculty size grew from 17,000 in 1965, to 39,000 in 1975, to 45,000 in 1978—an almost threefold increase in thirteen years. Biomedical research funding had little effect on the expansion in faculty size, however, for during those years biomedical research support was quite constant; it was probably due to increases in state and local funds for education and in revenues from professional fees and service programs.

It is of interest that, *at the level of the department,* differences in faculty size among schools does relate to differences in the support of research by the NIH. Dependence on federal biomedical research funds for faculty salaries varies; those institutions that have been successful in competing for NIH grants are more reliant on this source. One trend, according to the panel, is greater reliance on practice earnings for salaries of clinical faculty.

When the panel focused its attention on individual medical school departments it found universally what is known to everyone who has ever been a departmental chairman: they act as entrepreneurial units whose functions depend on their ability to generate funds from outside sources, tuition, capitation, and research. Because of this, according to the panel's report, departments may be quite vulnerable to cutbacks in research funding, and the parent institution may not have the flexibility to compensate them for such losses. Given the state of academic medical centers vis-à-vis research funding, two questions raised by the panel and by the AAMC should occupy our attention:

• Will medical schools be able to continue to attract creative young faculty members if funds for basic research continue to shrink?

• Will academic careers continue to attract creative young physicians if research and teaching programs continue to be diluted by requirements to engage in fund-generating patient care activities?

NIH SUPPORT FOR DEPARTMENTS OF PEDIATRICS AND CHILDREN'S HOSPITALS

The NIH is the major source of research funding for academic medical institutions. Funds from the NIH to departments of pediatrics and children's hospitals more than doubled between 1968 and 1979, expanding from 920 projects funded at about $41 million, to 1,076 projects funded at over $108 million (Table 3). In terms of real purchasing power, adjusted for inflation, however, the amount has barely increased over the years: translated into 1968 constant dollars, the 1979 total would amount to only about $52 million.

NIH support of pediatrics needs to be considered within the context of its total research budget, however. Figure 3, which is based on 1978 figures, shows the percentage to departments of pediatrics to be 3.1; that to obstetrics and gynecology, 0.7; and that to internal medicine, 5.4. It is important to note that these three departments received only 9.2

TABLE 3. SUPPORT OF DEPARTMENTS OF PEDIATRICS AND
CHILDREN'S HOSPITALS BY THE NATIONAL INSTITUTES OF HEALTH,
FISCAL YEARS 1969 TO 1979
(In Thousands of Dollars)

1968	$ 41,155
1969	43,346
1970	39,874
1971	45,304
1972	56,612
1973	56,041
1974	69,271
1975	74,906
1976	91,022
1977	83,750
1978	91,001
1979	108,371

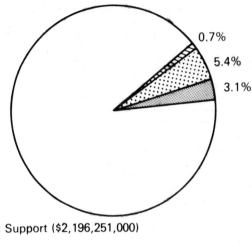

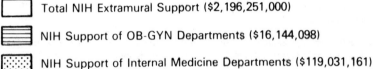

Total NIH Extramural Support ($2,196,251,000)

NIH Support of OB-GYN Departments ($16,144,098)

NIH Support of Internal Medicine Departments ($119,031,161)

NIH Support of Pediatrics Departments ($67,802,893)

Figure 3. Support of selected medical school departments in the United States by the National Institutes of Health, fiscal year 1978. The data do not include children's hospitals.

percent of the total, which indicates that NIH support is broad in gauge, cutting across many departments and disciplines.

Institutes within the NIH That Support Academic Pediatrics

Within the NIH the NICHD is the chief supporter of academic pediatrics, funding research activities in departments of pediatrics and children's hospitals at a level of $28.8 million in 1979 (Table 4).

The NICHD has been the leader throughout its history. In 1979 it was followed by the National Heart, Lung, and Blood Institute (NHLBI) at $22 million; the National Cancer Institute (NCI) at $19 million; and the National Institute of Arthritis, Metabolism, and Digestive Diseases (NIAMDD) at $13 million.

Nearly every institute of the NIH gives some support to research in academic pediatrics, but the content varies according to the mission of the institute. For example, the NCI funds

TABLE 4. SUPPORT OF DEPARTMENTS OF PEDIATRICS AND
CHILDREN'S HOSPITALS BY THE NATIONAL INSTITUTES OF HEALTH,
BY INSTITUTE, FISCAL YEARS 1968 AND 1979
(In Thousands of Dollars)

Institute	Fiscal Year 1968	Fiscal Year 1979
Child Health and Human Development	$10,038	$28,839
Heart, Lung, and Blood	4,361	22,139
Cancer	3,323	18,992
Arthritis, Metabolism, and Digestive Diseases	4,847	12,982
Allergy and Infectious Diseases	3,809	9,896
Division of Research Resources	8,866	5,636
General Medical Sciences	1,086	2,998
Neurological and Communicative Disorders and Stroke	4,634	2,646
Other NIH sources[1]	192	4,242

NOTE: 1) Institutes: Aging, Dental Research, Environmental Health Sciences, and Eye;
Fogarty International Center; National Library of Medicine.

research primarily concerned with cancer diagnosis and treatment in children; the NHLBI is most concerned with cardiac,
blood, and pulmonary problems of children; and the NIAMDD
focuses on juvenile diabetes, cystic fibrosis, and to some extent
juvenile arthritis.

Data from 1970–80 indicate that support from the NICHD
has almost tripled; that from the NHLBI has increased five-
fold; that from the NCI has increased sixfold; and that from the
NIAMDD has tripled. It is not so surprising that support of
pediatrics by the NCI and the NHLBI has grown by a greater
magnitude, given the dramatic increases in the budgets of those
two institutes during that decade. Yet in 1979 the NICHD
devoted 14.6 percent of its total budget to research in academic
pediatrics, whereas the NHLBI contributed only 4.3 percent,
and the NCI only 2 percent.

There is a great deal of concern currently about the types
of grants awarded to academic institutions and the mix of
granting mechanisms employed by the NIH. The President's
Biochemical Research Panel and the AAMC have expressed
concern about increasing reliance on large, program project
awards. Table 5 shows the mix of support instruments used by

TABLE 5. SUPPORT OF DEPARTMENTS OF PEDIATRICS AND
CHILDREN'S HOSPITALS BY THE NATIONAL INSTITUTES OF HEALTH,
BY MECHANISM, FISCAL YEARS 1968 AND 1979
(In Thousands of Dollars)

Mechanism	1968	1979
Research grants	$19,160	$54,535
Research projects	3,890	26,190
Research contracts	3,702	12,357
Training grants	5,678	4,640
Career development awards	2,104	2,973
Fellowships	741	1,030
Other NIH sources[1]	8,880	6,645

NOTE: 1) Refers to clinical research centers supported by the Division of Research Resources.

the NIH in departments of pediatrics and in children's hospitals, and how that mix has changed in the last decade.

Regular, investigator-initiated research grants and contracts increased almost threefold in dollar amounts between 1968 and 1979; program projects increased almost sevenfold. Research training grants, fellowships, and career development awards dropped in number and changed insignificantly in dollar amounts over the decade. When inflation is considered, however, the amount for the latter three mechanisms declines rather dramatically.

A Closer Look at Support from the NICHD

Within the NIH, the NICHD is the focal point for support of research in academic pediatrics. Figure 4 shows support from the NICHD to departments of pediatrics as a percentage of its total extramural budget. In 1978, 14.8 percent went to departments of pediatrics—a figure that would rise to about 15 percent if children's hospitals were included—compared to 6.6 percent to departments of obstetrics and gynecology.

Between 1968 and 1979 some rather dramatic changes occurred in NICHD support of pediatrics in terms of funding mechanisms. Table 6 indicates that funding for investigator-initiated research grants more than doubled in current dollars; program projects increased from five, funded at the level of $1.2 million, to twenty-four at almost $11 million; in 1979,

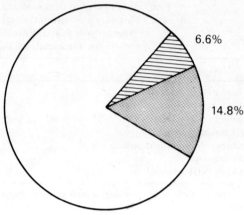

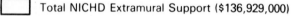

Total NICHD Extramural Support ($136,929,000)

Total NICHD Support to OB-GYN Departments ($8,977,923)

Total NICHD Support to Pediatrics Departments ($20,324,864)

Figure 4. Support of departments of pediatrics and of obstetrics and gynecology in the United States by the National Institute of Child Health and Human Development, fiscal year 1978. The data do not include children's hospitals.

twenty-two research contracts accounted for $2.3 million. Most important, training grants and career development awards dropped in both numbers and amounts awarded, and the total for fellowships stayed barely constant; in terms of constant dollars the amount actually dropped.

All mechanisms used by the NICHD are represented in the support of academic pediatrics, and they are utilized relatively

TABLE 6. SUPPORT OF DEPARTMENTS OF PEDIATRICS AND CHILDREN'S HOSPITALS
BY THE NATIONAL INSTITUTE OF CHILD HEALTH, AND HUMAN DEVELOPMENT,
BY MECHANISM, FISCAL YEARS 1968 AND 1979
(In Thousands of Dollars)

Mechanism	1968	1979
Research grants	$ 5,619	$13,618
Research projects	1,227	10,895
Research contracts	—	2,277
Training grants	2,037	1,214
Career development awards	976	647
Fellowships	179	187
Total NICHD support	$10,038	$28,838

evenly. The question of what is the proper mix of mechanisms to support a viable research endeavor is increasingly occupying the NIH and its individual institutes. These issues, particularly the decrease in funding for research training, should be of even greater concern to both the NIH and the academic medical institutions as total NIH appropriations level off in the next few years.

In years when research funding slows, another issue is raised—the likelihood of a well-designed, important research grant application not being funded. This has important implications, not only for the individual applicant, but for the department. As was pointed out earlier, departments act as entrepreneurs, and thus they can suffer if federal research funds drop off because departmental grant applications fail to compete well for support. The perception that only a small proportion of approved applications are funded can have devastating long-term effects if young people turn away from research careers on the ground that only a few can succeed.

In 1978, 62 percent of all types of applications from departments of pediatrics referred to the NICHD were approved, compared with 73 percent from departments of obstetrics and gynecology. Of those approved in pediatrics, 32 percent were funded. This is a respectable percentage, given that the average funding rate for all applications approved by the NICHD is about 22 percent. This figure is of course dependent on both the quality of the applications and the total appropriations available to the institute.

Research Training

When the President's Biomedical Research Panel prepared its report in 1976, one of its subpanels, referring to research training, wrote that

> . . . if there is to be a future for biomedical research in this country . . . the problem is the next generation of young scientists, who must be here and at work within the next decade. As things stand, the emergence of this generation is still a matter of doubt . . . . From the point of view of the youngest people, those just entering scientific careers and those just behind them trying to make up their minds, the future of biomedical science looks bleak indeed. The whole system seems to have become

abruptly locked up. Something will have to be done about this situation now or we will discover sometime in the 1980's that we have skipped a generation. . . . The scientific enterprise cannot undergo such a loss without serious damage to the future quality of research. It is not widely enough recognized that the youngest people, the ones still in training, are indispensable; they are not only essential for the future, they are also indispensable for the work that is being done today.[8]

The history of support for training by the NIH had its beginning in 1930, when the authority for training biomedical researchers was first given to the NCI. Between 1938 and 1972 the NIH contributed to the training of approximately 94,000 scientists, a major segment of the nation's biomedical research personnel. Funding peaked in 1969, when obligations totaled $168 million; it declined when support for research training was being phased out of most federal programs and when the NIH program came under question by the administration. The president's budget for fiscal year 1974 proposed a phasing out of ongoing training programs and termination of all new NIH training grants and fellowships on the ground that the nation faced a potential oversupply of scientific investigators; particularly under scrutiny was the training of clinical investigators. Congress strongly opposed subsidizing trainees who would later, presumably, enter clinical practice where the earning potential is high.

Passage of the 1974 National Research Service Award Act *authorized* training programs for the NIH and the Alcohol, Drug Abuse, and Mental Health Administration. A very important aspect of the law was the involvement of the National Academy of Sciences (NAS), which was to conduct a continuing study of the national need for biomedical and behavioral research personnel and determine the numbers and kinds of individuals to be trained. Thus the authority of the NIH to offer research training or fellowships in any given discipline came to depend on recommendations by the NAS.

Over the years the single most important factor that has depressed research training has been the gradual leveling off of NIH appropriations and the concomitant pressures imposed by increasing inflation. This effect can be seen in the amount of training funds flowing to pediatric departments over the years from the NIH as a whole, and from the NICHD in particular. NIH support for training in pediatrics dropped in current dollars between 1968 and 1979, with a slight recovery in 1973 and 1974. The NICHD witnessed a similar decline over the years, but it was far greater in terms of percentage of decrease: in the period 1975–80, the NIH as a whole had a 1 percent decline, compared with an 8.4 percent decline for the NICHD (Table 7).

For 1980 and 1981, at least, the picture for institutional research training grants and for fellowships does not look any brighter. A NIH-wide emphasis on investigator-initiated research grants—"stabilization"—at a time when the budget is staying essentially level means that other components of the NIH mix of support mechanisms will have to suffer the consequences. Moreover, for fiscal year 1980 the NIH put into effect a significant increase in stipends for individual and institutional trainees.

Because this action was implemented *after* the 1980 budget was constructed, the NICHD, for example, has had to establish policies that would accommodate a 31 percent increase in stipends within a budget about equal to that of fiscal year 1979. Because the NICHD has decided to cope with this situation by maintaining in all types of training programs the same number of trainees that were supported in 1979, there will be very little or no increase in training grants this year; the same seems to

TABLE 7. SUPPORT FOR TRAINING IN DEPARTMENTS OF PEDIATRICS AND CHILDREN'S HOSPITALS BY THE NATIONAL INSTITUTES OF HEALTH (NIH) AND THE NATIONAL INSTITUTE OF CHILD HEALTH AND HUMAN DEVELOPMENT (NICHD), FISCAL YEARS 1975 TO 1980
(In Thousands of Dollars)

	NIH	NICHD
1975	$ 6,864	$ 2,301
1976	6,260	2,131
1977	5,245	1,723
1978	5,803	1,740
1979	5,670	1,401
1980 (Estimated)	6,500	1,400
Total support	$36,342	$10,696

apply to fiscal year 1981. Over the years the proportion of NICHD funds awarded for training has been decreasing—from a high of 21 percent in 1967 to a low of 5 percent in 1979.

It is difficult to predict just what effect this curtailment of training funds will have on departments of pediatrics; some of them may have the mechanisms and resources to cope, at least temporarily, with shortfalls. In a recent study the National Research Council (NRC) concluded that curtailment of training funds affects the quality of training, that is, the important contribution of the research environment, as well as the number of persons in training.[9] It could be predicted that cutbacks in institutional training grants might have a greater effect on departmental operations than curtailments of individual fellowships. These institutional-type training grants provide support for programs, which, while based in one department, are multidisciplinary or interdisciplinary in scope. In addition to student stipends, tuition, and fees, a sum is provided to the department for the continuing enrichment of the research environment to assure the high quality of the experience.

Identified Areas of Need: Clinical Investigators

A clear shortage exists of clinical investigators with the M.D., D.D.S., D.V.M., or equivalent professional degree, and rigorous research training. This need has been recognized by the NIH, the NAS, and the AAMC.[10] In 1970 there were approximately 4,700 *clinical* postdoctoral fellows in research training positions, a figure that had dropped to approximately 1,800 in 1978; this is some 1,000 short of the recommendation of the NAS/NRC.

To try to correct this deficiency, the NICHD and other components of the NIH have recently announced a new clinical investigator award. This award, sought by the NICHD in pediatrics, clinical nutrition, obstetrics and gynecology, reproductive biology, and andrology, is expressly to help develop research ability in individuals with clinical backgrounds and training, rather than to further the development of research skills in individuals who have already demonstrated significant research achievement. Support is for three years, at a salary not to exceed $30,000 annually.

The purpose of the NIH training programs is to assure the continuance of a cadre of scientists of the highest quality to carry out the country's research programs. A critical mass of research trainees is the keystone of the biomedical research endeavor. In my view the whole health care system of the country will stagnate without the supply of fresh ideas, coupled with dedication and enthusiasm.

CONCLUSION

From this discussion of current perspectives in pediatrics and federal support of academic pediatrics, I believe three major themes have emerged that will continue, at least for the next several years, to have great impact on the future of academic pediatrics. These three trends—entrenchment of specialization, heavier reliance on funds from clinical services, and a leveling off of federal research support, particularly training support—affect all branches of academic medicine, not just pediatrics. But pediatrics, as mentioned earlier, has always been a field that has responded to social currents, and the leaders in pediatrics have always had a penchant for examining and reflecting on the state of their discipline and the political, social, and economic factors that affect it. It is my hope that the giants of today's pediatrics will take the lead among medical academicians and work to shape the pediatrics of tomorrow, rather than allow currents to carry it helter skelter.

NOTES

1. T. E. Cone, Jr., *History of American Pediatrics* (Boston: Little, Brown, 1979).

2. L. E. Holt, "American Pediatrics—A Retrospect and a Forecast," *Transactions of the American Pediatric Society* 35 (21 May–2 June 1973): 9–17.

3. William Osler, "Remarks on Specialism," *Transactions of the American Pediatric Society* 4 (2–4 May 1892): 6–13.

4. W. H. Steward, "The Unmet Needs of Children," *Pediatrics* 39 (February 1976): 159–60.

5. *Medical Education: Institutions, Characteristics, and Programs, A Background Paper* (Washington: Association of American Medical Colleges, August 1976).

6 American Council on Education, Association of American Medical Colleges, and the Rand Corporation, "Appendix C: Impact of Federal Health-Related Expenditures upon Institutions of Higher Education," in *Report of the President's Biomedical Research Panel*, DHEW publication no. (OS) 76-503 (Bethesda Maryland: Department of Health, Education, and Welfare, 30 April 1976).

7. Department of Health and Human Services, *Basic Data Relating to the National Institutes of Health,* NIH publication no. 80-1261 (Bethesda, Maryland: National Institutes of Health, March 1980).

8. *President's Panel* (See note 6).

9. Commission on Human Resources, *Personnel Needs and Training for Biomedical and Behavioral Research* (Washington: National Research Council, 1979).

10. Ad Hoc Committee of the Association of American Medical Colleges, "A Policy for Biomedical and Behavioral Research," *Journal of Medical Education* 54 (March 1979): 259–73.

DISCUSSANT:

Floyd W. Denny

Kretchmer has presented the perspectives of academic pediatrics relative to history, content, personnel, and federal financial support. As a pediatric departmental chairman, I should like to talk about some of the greatest challenges that face academic pediatrics in the immediate future. In my opinion these challenges include the overall financial support of our departments; the entry of young academicians into our subspecialty; and a continuing and adequate source of patients for teaching and research purposes. Financial support and manpower supply will be touched on briefly; I shall go into more detail about the availability of patients.

Funding of the day-by-day operations of the department is probably the greatest problem faced by most pediatric chairmen. This problem is not confined to pediatrics, of course, but we are probably the hardest hit of the clinical departments because the discipline is traditionally the least affluent of the subspecialties. While most of us are attempting to solve at least some of our problems by increasing our time and effectiveness in the practice of pediatrics, I seriously doubt that this will prove to be an adequate answer. I envision any great surge in private practice as being a destructive influence on academic excellence.

The financing of academic pediatrics must be faced by academic medicine as a whole, and we must be joined by other subspecialties in solving this dilemma. I do not want to sound too pessimistic; after a few years of austerity I am confident we shall overcome our financial difficulties. Since I have no ready answers I shall not pursue the subject further.

The assurance of an adequate supply of young academicians entering pediatrics may be the most serious long-range problem. The reasons for this are many, probably extremely complicated, and certainly not restricted to pediatrics. The following factors play roles to varying degrees in this matter:

• Societal pressure to practice clinical medicine.
• The salary differential between academic medicine and practice.
• The long training required for academicians.
• Difficulties in obtaining research funding.
• Lack of job opportunities in academic pediatrics.
• The attractiveness of other intellectual disciplines.

The fact that pediatric practitioners are usually paid considerably less than other medical subspecialties probably will help us in this regard. I have no ready and easy solutions to the manpower issue, but we must keep it in mind constantly and keep working on it if we are to survive.

The question I want to consider in most detail is the source of patients for teaching and research purposes. In doing so I am going to make the assumption that departments of pediatrics in this country will remain the cornerstone of teaching and research in the field of children's health and medical care. That is not to say of course that departments of family medicine, maternal and child health, child psychiatry and psychology, and various surgical subspecialties do not play important roles.

But departments of pediatrics remain the hub of the pediatric teaching and research wheel.

In discussing health and medical care it is convenient and customary to separate the levels of care into tertiary, or care in a referral hospital; secondary, or care in a community hospital; and primary, or ambulatory care. I shall give a bit of past history, assess the present status, and attempt to predict the future in each of these areas.

The types of patients on a pediatric teaching service are in a state of great and rapid change. Twenty to thirty years ago our wards were filled with children with pneumonia, diarrhea, meningitis, poliomyelitis, diphtheria, pertussis, and tetanus. Now a large proportion are in neonatal intensive care units, and other beds are filled with children with cancer, organ transplants, congenital defects, and major genetic disorders. This radical change has been brought about by multiple factors. Many communicable diseases can now be prevented by vaccines or improved methods of sanitation, and antibiotics control many bacterial infections. Another factor, however, is that in some ways we are the victims of our own successes. Children who several years ago would have been cared for in a tertiary hospital are now being treated in community hospitals, or even on an ambulatory basis.

This brings us to the changes taking place in secondary care, which in many ways are more radical than those just mentioned. Only a few years ago there were few pediatricians outside major metropolitan areas, and there were few, if any, pediatric beds in community hospitals; in 1980 excellent pediatricians are practicing in very fine community hospitals. Hospitalization in such services has many attractive features, including the proximity to the children's homes, lower costs, and the absence of the distractions and annoyances caused by the presence of house staff and students. Moreover, in North Carolina we have the impression that the alarming increases in transportation costs represent another large factor.

The nature of ambulatory care in pediatrics is also changing, although probably to a lesser degree than in other areas. Kretchmer has mentioned the increasing emphasis on developmental, behavioral, and social sciences in pediatric care. The use of pediatric nurse practitioners or associates is also causing some changes, but probably not as much as it should. The provision of pediatric care through health maintenance organizations or other prepaid plans has had an effect, and in some parts of the country the health and medical care provided through local health departments is a major factor.

What, then, are the big issues presented by the radical changes taking place in the primary, secondary, and tertiary care of children? Here again I make the assumption that it is not only desirable but absolutely necessary for academic pediatrics to play a large part in teaching and research at all three levels of patient care. I should like to address these problems in the same order as they have just been presented.

In my opinion academic pediatric services must be the ultimate in the care of sick children, and as such must be at the cutting edge of the application of new therapeutic measures. This means our neonatal intensive care units must continue to be developed; intensive care units for older children must be improved; transplantation and dialysis units must play a large part in our everyday life; complicated cancer treatment should continue to be developed; and we should be constantly introducing newer knowledge in our care of children who have immunological, genetic, and pharmacological problems.

If these measures are carried out as well as they should be, an entirely new set of problems arise. Wards filled with such patients are not ideal as the sole source of teaching material for medical students or pediatric house staff, most of whom still want to practice general pediatrics. Although such patients are ideal for certain types of teaching and research, we need a greater spectrum of patients to do the job well.

I do not believe anything can or should be done to deter the provision of excellent pediatric care in community hospitals. It is imperative, however, that these patients be incorporated into our teaching and research plans. Attempts to do this have brought about, and will continue to bring about, a new set of problems. Geographic separation from our academic institutions is a serious issue, but probably relatively minor compared to such factors as the quality control of teaching and acceptance by practicing pediatricians and the public.

The biggest problem we are facing and shall continue to face is finding sufficient patients for teaching and research purposes in the primary care area. Most health and medical care is given to children outside hospitals, and ambulatory care makes up the greatest part of any pediatrician's practice. It seems to me that most of the activities of practitioners of pediatrics are based on empiricism; there are far too few facts to guide us in the provision of health and medical care. Unfortunately, research in this area is difficult to conduct, expensive, frequently takes years to complete, and requires skills that few pediatricians have learned. In spite of such obstacles, we must attack these problems vigorously.

It is important now to attempt to draw the three levels of patient care into a coherent whole for a comprehensive health care system for children. It is certain that primary, secondary, and tertiary care must all be given consideration if the services given to children are to be efficient, cost effective, and medically acceptable. Furthermore, I am convinced that the regionalization of medical care and the provision of care by nurse practitioners and other professionals, in addition to the physician, are necessary and desirable developments that will be instituted in the future. I am convinced also that if academic pediatrics does not lead the way in these endeavors, some other force, notably the federal government, will dictate our future course.

In summary, I have attempted to outline the perspectives of a pediatric departmental chairman in terms of funding, manpower, and a source of patients for teaching and research purposes. All three present problems that are important, but greatest emphasis is placed on the last issue. It appears that radical changes are taking place in the quality of patients available to academic medicine at all levels of care. If we are going to continue to be leaders in the teaching of pediatrics and in research on the health and medical care needs of children, it is essential that we be responsive to these changes in every way possible.

PRIVATE FOUNDATIONS AND
THE FUTURE OF ACADEMIC PEDIATRICS

Robert J. Haggerty

I will report on three aspects of pediatrics in this presentation. First, the funding of pediatric departments: in preparation for this meeting I undertook a survey of the 128 administrative divisions of medical schools in the United States in which I asked about the funding of their departments of pediatrics and the changes in sources of money that had occurred over the last five years; second, I will review the major findings of the Carnegie Commission on Children, especially those relating to health; and, finally, I will summarize some of my own views about the role of private foundations in the future of pediatrics in the United States.

SURVEY OF CURRENT FUNDING
OF PEDIATRIC DEPARTMENTS

In response to the brief questionnaire sent to the medical schools seventy-seven completed responses were received—twenty-four from private medical schools and fifty-three from state-supported institutions. (Detailed tables appear in the appendix to this chapter). From these data, and from discussions of the results of the survey with members of the Association of Pediatric Department Chairmen at its annual meeting, several conclusions are apparent:

- There is an extraordinary diversity in the sources of support of American medical schools—especially perhaps of

departments of pediatrics—which vary from small, generally
new, state institutions, in which up to 100 percent of all their
resources, which may amount to less than $250,000 a year,
come from the parent university, to one private medical school
with an annual pediatric faculty budget of nearly $9 million,
most of which comes from federal research funds. In general,
state schools receive much more of their support from the
university than do the private, independent schools.

• The largest increase in sources of funds in the past five
years has derived from the service sector—from hospital revenues and physicians' fees for services. This is regarded with
considerable concern by many, since it cuts into the time available to the faculty for teaching and research; in pediatrics,
especially, with a relatively low reimbursement rate per hours
spent, this is a significant deterrent for young faculty members
to pursue academic careers.

• Fellowship programs are concentrated in a very few
schools. There are somewhere between 900 and 1,000 fellow
positions available in the United States, but only about 600 of
them are filled. One institution has 119 fellows in residence at
present. Some schools have more than ten fellows, but the vast
majority have fewer than ten. Fellowships usually represent the
source of new faculty. It is certainly safe to say that few schools,
perhaps ten to a dozen at most, train the majority of subspecialists and future faculty.

• There is considerable variety in reimbursement plans for
full-time faculty in those schools that are still strictly full time
and in others that have a base salary with unlimited supplements. In view of the rapid increase in private practice plans, it
is surprising that there is still a strict full-time system in a
considerable number of schools. The questionnaire did not tap
the degree of satisfaction or dissatisfaction with various salary
plans, but it is clear from discussions with faculty members that
this is a source of considerable tension in many institutions. Full
or strict full-time systems often lead to a lack of incentive to
recapture fees for services rendered, and to discontent among
faculty who perceive considerable differences in their responsibility for patient care and yet receive the same salary. On the
other hand, some schools with a base salary permit such large

increases from practice plans that the discrepancy between high-earning and low-earning faculty creates serious imbalances within the department and the school.

• A final question asked for suggestions as to needs. The responses ranged over almost the entire spectrum of departmental activities, but clearly the two most commonly reported sources were: a) support for new faculty members, especially for time spent on research, to help them avoid too great a burden of patient care during this critical period; and b) support for certain special fellowships. Traditional fellowships are reasonably well-supported, but fellowships in ambulatory, behavioral, and general pediatrics face difficulties because patient care and research sources are less available for these areas.

RECOMMENDATIONS OF THE CARNEGIE COMMISSION ON CHILDREN

The Carnegie Commission, whose mission was to consider the needs of children generally, was made up of individuals from a variety of backgrounds; I was the only one from the health arena. While health received a considerable amount of attention, and it is the subject of one chapter of the report, it is only one of the many aspects of children's needs that were identified by the commission.

Initially, a considerable amount of discussion developed between what might be called the "service-oriented" members of the commission and those with the "money-jobs" approach. Another way to characterize this division of opinion might be to call the former the "micro," or individual or small group approach, versus the "macro," or social policy, approach. After a great deal of discussion and weighing of the evidence the commission as a whole opted in its primary recommendations to support the macro approach. It was felt that without jobs and a basic floor of income for families it would be difficult for children to benefit from most of the other services that were being recommended, such as education, social services, and health care.

In part this recommendation was based on the fact that, increasingly, society is becoming convinced that provision of health services, even when heretofore they may have been minimal or nonexistent, can make only a marginal improvement in the level of health of children as a group. In contrast, an adequate income and jobs for the parents are necessary not only to meet daily needs for food, clothing, and shelter, but to provide motivation for the children. Only when they see their parents employed will most children realize that meaningful work will be available to them as adults. In the long run this may have a greater impact, even on health, than health services alone.

The recommendations contained several specific characteristics of a desirable health service for children. These included proposals that:

• Nonmedical influences should be made an integral part of the health care system.

• Barriers to access be removed.

• Services for children emphasize preventive and humane, as well technological, care.

• Publicly accountable child health agencies be created in each area to administer and supervise these services.

• As part of the health services, attention be paid to increasing the capacity of parents and children to act on their own behalf as advocates and as self-caretakers in the health arena.

The implication for pediatrics is that, in general, private foundations will in the future be less interested in narrow medical approaches to improving the health of populations of children; at the very least, joint efforts with other disciplines will be necessary. There also needs to be a greater emphasis on preventive medicine, health education, and promotion of good health habits—areas that in the past have generally not had a high priority.

THE ROLE OF PRIVATE FOUNDATIONS IN ACADEMIC PEDIATRICS

As one of the "new boys" in the foundation world it would be presumptuous of me to speak for the some 25,000 private foundations in the United States. I will, however, summarize some of the conclusions reached by a group of "health grant makers" representing several of the larger foundations with an interest in health who met in Dallas on 28 May 1980:

• Everyone agreed that there will be a drastic retrenchment in social investment, especially in health services, in the 1980s.

• The available public dollars will be used to provide for already mandated services, rather than to add on new ones.

• Corporate funds will increasingly join with private foundations to support innovations.

• Private foundation support, although small in comparison to state and federal monies, will represent an important resource for innovation.

Two major areas of need were recognized that will probably be of interest to foundations in terms of possible support. The first is how individuals can be taught self-care and preventive habits that will improve health and decrease demands on health care services. Second, there will be a shift in support of some manpower training programs from the concern of the past decade about increasing the number of primary care practitioners to attention to the needs of research-oriented faculty, minorities, and academic primary care. Research-oriented faculty, especially in primary care, will be in short supply. In addition, it will be difficult to support new faculty; a lack of new money, retirement at a later age, and many departments filled with relatively young tenured faculty will make it very difficult for new young faculty to advance during the 1980s. This situation will be especially acute in behavioral and general medicine. Private foundations will probably respond to requests in these two areas with greater interest than in some of the traditional disease-oriented areas.

If pediatrics departments respond to what is perceived by foundations as creative and innovative approaches to major problems, foundations in turn will provide help with start-up, evaluation, and developmental funds. There will also be increasing coordination of the efforts of groups of foundations, including industrial foundations, which will join together to support various aspects of projects. They will together seek to influence federal policies to carry on the funding of programs demonstrated to be effective. Private foundations cannot be looked to as sources of support for existing programs that face declining sources of funding.

APPENDIX

QUESTIONNAIRE SENT TO
128 ADMINISTRATIVE DIVISIONS OF
AMERICAN MEDICAL SCHOOLS CONCERNING
RESOURCES OF DEPARTMENTS OF PEDIATRICS
SUMMARY OF RESPONSES FROM 77 SCHOOLS

I. Approximately what proportion of the income of your faculty, as a whole, derives from:

	Percentages			
	75–100	50–75	25–50	0–25
STATE SCHOOLS				
University	9	23	15	6
Research				
Federal	—	—	4	49
Other	—	—	—	53
Services				
Hospital	—	2	4	47
Patient care	—	1	12	40
Other			4	40
PRIVATE AND INDEPENDENT SCHOOLS				
University	1	2	5	16
Research				
Federal	—	1	4	19
Other	—	—	3	21
Services				
Hospital	4	1	3	16
Patient care	—	1	6	17
Other	—	1	1	22

APPENDIX (Continued)

II. Size of departments of pediatrics

	Number of Faculty Members						
	10	10–20	20–30	30–40	40–50	50–75	75+
STATE SCHOOLS	4	17	11	9	6	4	2
PRIVATE AND INDEPENDENT SCHOOLS	1	1	7	6	3	2	4

	Number of House Staff					
	10	10–20	20–30	30–40	40–50	50+
STATE SCHOOLS	4	13	10	13	6	7
PRIVATE AND INDEPENDENT SCHOOLS	1	1	4	8	2	8

	Number of Fellows					
STATE SCHOOLS	29	12	4	2	3	3
PRIVATE AND INDEPENDENT SCHOOLS	10	7	2	2	1	1

III. What is the status of your full-time faculty?

	State Schools	Private and Independent Schools
Strict full-time, with no supplementation permitted	17	9
Base salary plus predetermined supplement	15	3
Base salary plus supplement up to a maximum figure	19	12
Base salary plus unlimited supplements	2	—

APPENDIX (Continued)

IV. Size of departmental budget, 1979–80

	Faculty Only	
	State Schools	Private and Independent Schools
$250,000 or less	4	2
$250,000–$500,000	4	1
$500,000–$750,000	9	1
$750,000–$1 million	9	2
$1–2 million	13	8
$2–3 million	11	3
$3 million or more	3	7

	Research			
	Federal	Other	Federal	Other
$250,000 or less	15	12	4	7
$250–500,000	4	5	5	4
$500–750,000	3	4	2	1
$750,000–$1 million	7	5	1	2
$1–2 million	8	5	3	3
$2–3 million	4	2	3	1
$3 million or more	—	—	2	2

MODELS OF ACADEMIC PEDIATRICS

MODELS OF ACADEMIC PEDIATRICS: TRAINING IN THE MEDICAL SCHOOLS

Joseph W. St. Geme, Jr.

Pediatrics has probably suffered no more than other disciplines in the wake of: 1) the federal redirection of the academic mission; 2) the extraordinary sense of national pragmatism; and 3) the relative inflationary gallop of our economy during the past several years. Internal medicine, probably the most consistent and visible bastion of the academic spirit, has possibly fared somewhat better. But even the elite internists, threatened by the emergence of family practice, have diverted considerable energy to the realignment of forces from subspecialty adult medicine to the rediscovery of primary care. The other major discipline, surgery, has responded to the trumpeting of provocative faculty practice plans and strict full-time academic salaries with an almost lethal self-dissolution of the rich heritage of surgical science and scholarship. Family practice is just beginning to develop an academic base. Unfortunately, however, the critical mass of faculty is somewhat out of synchrony with the rapid proliferation of great numbers of undergraduate and postgraduate educational programs. Elaborating this personal perspective and introduction somewhat further, may I suggest that obstetrics and gynecology continue to tread water in the academic stream. This may be considered to represent relative progress. We can all do so much better!

ROLE MODELS FOR STUDENTS

Let us look at academic pediatrics. Let us look at the role models for our bright young medical students and residents. Our pediatrics faculties have increased in great numbers throughout the United States during the past quarter-century and more. After World War II, during the halcyon days of the National Institutes of Health under the remarkable direction of James A. Shannon, and with the resolute support of Lister Hill of Alabama and John E. Fogarty of Rhode Island and their willing colleagues in Congress, there evolved a fresh explosion of scientific medicine and an almost unparalleled opportunity for the development of aspiring, inquiring young academic pediatricians, cut in the Oslerian mode of teacher-investigator-clinician-scholar. Spirits were keen, sound dollars were available, and the professional lifestyle of the academician was exhilarating.

In the mid-1960s the rapidly evolving steeples of excellence in academic pediatrics began to sway in the turbulent winds of regional medical programs, comprehensive community health centers, the new jargon of health care systems, and governmental exhortations to translate fundamental discoveries very quickly into meaningful clinical care.

Academic pediatrics, always a marginal economic operation, began to confront a quickly broadening spectrum of new, and diluting, challenges and the temptation of Willie Sutton's Law, that is, "go where the money is." For fifteen years academic pediatrics departments have struggled to maintain the balanced trilogy of teaching, research, and patient care. In far too many departments, research, always a tough competitive process, has been dispatched to the arena of faint hope and supplanted by an enormous array of health care operations, primary, secondary, and tertiary in nature. These health care operations were designed to compete with a growing population of skilled general and consultative pediatricians in small or large group practices.

More recently, pediatrics faculties have *added* to the energy-depleting enterprise of perinatal and neonatal intensive care—which, parenthetically, have become so highly successful—the vast and important ambulatory care components of emergency medicine, adolescent medicine, and behavioral pediatrics. As has been true of perinatal-neonatal medicine, during the past decade more attention has been devoted to *doing the work* than to *asking the questions*. Presumably the academic pediatrician is better prepared and motivationally suited to a life of inquiry than is the practicing pediatric clinician. One might conclude, unhappily, that the zeal and excitement of the quest for knowledge in all these new, as well as traditional, fields of pediatrics does *not* engulf every academic pediatrics department in this country.

Joy and enthusiasm about one's professional life, whether academic or clinical, are the ingredients that seem to entice a substantial number of students to a similar career decision. Role models in our medical schools, men and women who can share the experience of clinical perspectives of pediatrics and a dynamic sense of the exploration of the biomedical frontiers in our field, draw the greatest number of younger men and women to academic pediatrics. Assuming for the moment that we have a reasonably balanced supply of triple-threat pediatric academicians, that is, individuals who are able to teach, conduct research, provide care, and excite students—an enormous assumption—the curricula in our medical schools and teaching hospitals should provide ample opportunity to attract some of our finest young minds and spirits to academic pediatrics.

Drawing on the second and third years of undergraduate education, with six to nine weeks of instruction we have sufficient time to introduce students to the particulars of the history taking and physical examination of the infant, child, and perhaps even the adolescent. We also have enough time to emphasize the dynamic elements of perinatal adaptation, developmental kinetics, and human growth. If undue emphasis is placed on an extended ambulatory experience one risks the presentation of a fragmented, superficial, expeditious, albeit exciting notion of pediatrics.

CLERKSHIPS

On the other hand, the well-organized junior student clerkship, which maximizes significant responsibility and participation on an inpatient ward service team, presents a magnificent Oslerian opportunity to learn data retrieval in depth; diagnosis; the essentials but not the specific details of care; the fundamentals of the pathophysiology and the pathogenesis of the illnesses of infants and children; a host of exciting and important behavioral issues that surround almost every hospitalized child; and, most critically important, the constantly evolving link between the dynamic, complex, basic sciences and clinical medicine.

The traditional ward clerkship, a closely knit team of students and residents, skilled faculty teaching and supervision, fresh, challenging clinical problems, and readily available, but restrained, consultative subspecialists supply the essential ingredients for learning, excitement, and successful seduction into academic pediatrics. And for this next decade, we need to seduce the very best!

The neonatal intensive care unit may be too swift and sophisticated an environment for the junior medical student. The evolving intermediate care unit in our teaching hospitals, however, which now deals with high-risk term and preterm infants and a broad spectrum of provocative perinatal issues, comfortable even for the nonneonatologist academician to address, represents an excellent setting for contemporary learning, intellectual stimulation, and the ultimate focusing of inquisitive young minds on the very best of modern pediatrics.

The junior clerkship and the senior advanced clerkships, or subinternships, in general and subspecialty pediatrics, particularly in the general teaching hospital, present unique opportunities to work in interdisciplinary collaboration with almost the entire spectrum of clinical specialties, including internal medicine and obstetrics and gynecology. This is a very refreshing aspect of pediatrics, in contrast to so many other disciplines, and the young person with a broad perspective of scientific inquiry can find amplification of this sense of collaborative scholarship in the pediatric milieu.

The recent solidification of postgraduate pediatric residency training as a three-year curricular program has raised serious and responsible questions in the minds of some of our finest academic leaders. There is concern that the three-year general pediatric training requirement will deter aspirants from choosing a career in academic pediatrics. Implicit in this concern is the notion that the majority of recent academic aspirants pursued only two years of general pediatric training before entering subspecialty fellowship experiences designed, presumably, to prepare them for an academic career. Statistical analysis of this important point by the American Board of Pediatrics indicates that 90 percent of individuals who were able to take either two or three years of general pediatrics prior to fellowship training chose three years of general work. The number of pediatric fellows is estimated to be 1,000, but only 20 percent are believed to be pursuing a true academic career of significant, tough-minded research in addition to teaching and patient care.

POSTDOCTORAL FELLOWSHIPS

There exists at present, within the context of three years of general pediatric residency training, sufficient flexibility for the clearly committed resident to shift after two or two and a half years to a substantive, rigorous postdoctoral fellowship program designed, one hopes, to prepare her/him for a research-oriented academic career. The more significant time-frame problem in the postgraduate years, in my view, is *not* two versus three years of general pediatric training, but, in sharp contrast, the current predilection of so many fellowship program directors and trainees to devote only two years to this effort. Three years of disciplined scientific training are necessary to conduct consistent, imaginative, and successful biomedical research.

In the main, two-year fellows will drift within short order from junior faculty, clinically oriented academic posts to a hybrid of general and subspecialty pediatric practice. Although this does not represent a total failure, by the same token it does not offer an attractive focus for young students and young residents who attach more quickly to bright, exciting, and successful young faculty; nor does this course of events satisfy our great need for dynamic, creative new academic pediatricians.

Considering the stiff economic challenge of pursuing a third year of fellowship training, which represents the sixth year beyond graduation, some departments are beginning to offer transitional, research-oriented academic appointments with stipends that, while less than that of the usual assistant professor, exceed that of the traditional fellowship.

RESTRUCTURING PRIORITIES

The problem is not a new breed of students or residents. Curricula and students are returning to more traditional concepts of teaching and learning, retaining some of the best of the new horizons of the past decade. We, the academic pediatricians, are the problem. We must take the best of what has transpired during the past decade—and some of its dilutional diversions—and restructure our priorities. We are the most likely ones, perhaps the only ones, who can create new knowledge. Our business is research, development, and strategy, not wholesale tactics, as important as they are. Redirection of energy, improved organization, better collaboration, and imaginative interdisciplinary science can provide academic pediatrics departments with new force and vitality. A host of academic pediatric Pied Pipers scattered throughout the country will bring forth the ultimate harvest of a new wave of young talent from among our medical school undergraduate and postgraduate students in our teaching hospitals.

Academic pediatrics enjoys a rich and productive heritage of diversity and a broad commitment to the total preventive and therapeutic biomedical and psychosocial needs of children. Indeed we may have constructed the "mission impossible." No other academic clinical discipline attempts to do so much for so many with so little in the way of total resources—but of so much importance to our nation's future.

At the risk of continued hyperbole may I exhort academic pediatricians to review their spirit of inquiry and fundamental investigation at every step and branching path along the way of this challenging journey.

MODELS OF ACADEMIC PEDIATRICS: THE ROLE OF CHILDREN'S HOSPITALS

Mary Ellen Avery

I shall discuss the role of children's hospitals in academic pediatrics with emphasis on their suitability as sites for training medical students and house staff and as centers for research on child health and disease. I assume the reason this topic was assigned to me is that I have had the privilege of working in a children's hospital contiguous with a general hospital—the Johns Hopkins Hospital—and in two of the largest independent children's hospitals on this continent, the Montreal Children's Hospital and the Children's Hospital in Boston.

All three of these institutions, and I assume most other children's hospitals, were established by groups of individuals who joined forces to create an environment dedicated to the special needs of children. Often the prime movers were orthopedists who realized that youngsters confined to bed for many months needed special attention, such as school lessons, and that these requirements were not well met in general hospitals. Separate facilities for children may of course be provided as a part of a general hospital, as is the case at Johns Hopkins, the Massachusetts General Hospital and Bellevue Hospital in New York, where distinguished children's services do indeed exist in a setting where the majority of the beds and most of the staff are dedicated to the care of the adult.

I recognize the difficulty of making judgments about the quality of services, but if we reflect on the past it is fair to say

61

that many of the major contributions to the understanding of children's diseases have emanated from children's hospitals. The importance of research was recognized very early by such institutions as the Children's Hospital in Cincinnati, the Hospital for Sick Children in Toronto, Baltimore's Harriet Lane Home, and the children's hospitals in Boston, Philadelphia and Montreal, to name just a few. It is less easy to identify major contributions directed toward diseases of children that have emanated from the usually smaller pediatric wards of community or general hospitals.

RESEARCH CENTERS

On reflecting on the reasons for the primacy of children's hospitals as centers for pediatric research one can give credit to several trends. An obvious one is that an independent institution with its own board of trustees and fund-raising capacity can set aside endowment funds that serve the needs of children. The opening of research institutes in Cincinnati and Toronto helped foster research in both centers. The creation of laboratory space for investigators who came from the ranks of pediatrics and were concerned about diseases of children at the Harriet Lane Home, the Montreal Children's Hospital, and the Boston Children's Hospital gave institutional recognition to the independence of research and the quality of patient care. Another important factor in the establishment of academic programs in pediatrics is the close affiliation of the teaching hospitals with medical schools, and the participation of both university and hospital personnel in the appointment of all department or division heads in the hospitals. In institutions where there is a dichotomy in the medical leadership of the hospital and the university programs there is in general a less distinguished academic record, and in many respects a less satisfactory environment for patient care.

A consequence of the selection of appropriate medical school professors who also serve as key department heads in the children's hospitals has been the evolution and expansion of residency training programs and of the environment for teaching medical students in the hospital. A university has little interest in professors who are not involved in training at some level; the recruitment of outstanding faculty members hinges on their ability to attract outstanding students. The future of pediatrics depends on a high-quality and exciting academic enterprise in an appropriate milieu. The presence of a distinguished clinical faculty, in turn, greatly enhances patient care.

FELLOWSHIP PROGRAMS

The significant growth of the fellowship training program at the Boston Children's Hospital in recent years—119 fellows in pediatrics and its subspecialties in 1979–80—testifies to the thirst of a faculty for young people with whom to work, as well as the desire of postresidents to embark on two to three years of fellowship (or apprenticeship) in order to learn a subspecialty and acquire the research tools with which to advance the frontiers.

The total impact of fellowship programs is not always fully appreciated by most of the principals concerned, however. From the fellows' perspective they are embarking on a research and training expedition. They consider they have all the inherent rights and privileges of students, including access to good libraries, time dedicated to research, and the opportunity to teach. The fellows do not often take into consideration the costs of office and laboratory space, of supplies such as stationery, or of the use of telephones, dining facilities, common rooms, and even parking space. The fellows' view is that in providing some consultation services for patients and in teaching house staff they are paying in services for their part of the overhead.

From the point of view of the faculty, fellows become an amplifier for the conduct of research; in clinics and in laboratories they contribute immensely to the generation of new ideas. From the perspective of a department head, a certain number of fellows becomes a measure of the attractiveness of the academic program. When training grants or other extramural funds provide the fellows' salaries, when their research brings recognition, and when they teach and care for a few patients they can be regarded as one of the most valuable resources.

Some problems arise when fellows outnumber house

officers and when many of them want appointments to the faculty. A complex spiral emerges when their preceptors require more space for their expanding research needs, and when the fellows collectively claim more of the time and attention of their preceptors than does the house staff.

Should there be a limit to the number of fellows in each program? The possibility of a finite limit of course has an impact on the issue of the need for academicians, which in turn seems to have some sensitivity to the market place. Most of the subspecialties of pediatrics are still understaffed, so quotas have not been imposed by the regulatory agencies or by other sectors of society. The major limitation on numbers of fellows is the wish of the preceptors, their ability to attract financial support, and their perceptions of how to train investigators.

CHALLENGES

What are the arguments for expanding the academic thrust in children's hospitals? The central issue arises from recognition of major unsolved problems of childhood disorders, whose solutions are more likely to come from research associated with academic pediatric services than from other centers: many birth defects, for example, can best be studied in children's hospitals, as can inborn errors of metabolism, which include diseases such as cystic fibrosis, juvenile onset diabetes, and some forms of asthma. Many developmental dysfunctions are poorly understood, and this places strong demands on children's hospitals for further research on learning disabilities and the detection of other neurological disorders. One of the greatest challenges currently before us is to take advantage of recombinant DNA technology for the replacement of missing genes, and the production of gene products by such replacement. Surely these clinical interventions would have most meaning if carried out early in life—thus a children's hospital is a natural laboratory for clinical genetics.

Among the other challenges to academic pediatrics is the control of infectious diseases, which has an illustrious past—the development of immunization against poliomyelitis, for example—and an even more promising future when one contemplates the possibility of rapid viral diagnosis and the availability of virucidal agents. Identification of childhood precursors of adult illnesses is a continuing focus as we strive to establish our role as practitioners of preventive medicine.

SPECIAL NEEDS OF CHILDREN

I would be remiss if I failed to mention some of the other reasons why children's hospitals are excellent places to teach medical students, nurses, house staff, and other professionals concerned with children. One of the great strengths of an institution of several hundred beds that can support surgical subspecialty areas and ancillary services is that all individuals on the staff are sympathetic to the special needs of children. It is also evident that the ambience of most children's hospitals is pleasant; the attitudes of nurses, child-life workers, social workers, and others contribute toward a rather more attractive environment than is found in most adult institutions, as our students frequently note.

The special needs of certain kinds of children require the organization of learning centers, special schools, and other services that do such an outstanding job they become models for individuals who will eventually provide these services in other settings. In the children's hospitals with which I have been associated, individuals from many schools and colleges, including physical therapists, psychologists, audiologists, and various kinds of technicians come to acquire a facility in the pediatric aspects of their particular specialty. Thus the focus for learning applies not only to medical and nursing students, but to individuals concerned with all aspects of continuing education.

THE WARD AS CLASSROOM

The coexistence of an extensive teaching enterprise and patient care, often on the same crowded wards, is not without problems that deserve constant attention and resolution. Teaching within earshot of patients can be viewed as talking over their heads; rotating house officers disrupt continuity of care; the insecurity of younger staff may result in more laboratory tests than an experienced pediatrician would request; multiple consultants may transmit conflicting messages to patients and parents with consequent unnecessary anxiety; and, an often overlooked issue, the patient may get little rest amidst the turmoil of teachers and learners performing repeated examinations. Worst of all, when issues of poor communication do arise we hear rumblings about the need for patient advocates. I believe advocacy is the responsibility of the physician and the nurse, and I am troubled, in fact alarmed, that well-intentioned souls should presume to suggest the need for intermediaries between professionals and patients.

Among the obvious solutions to the problem of the ward as a classroom is the allocation of more space for teaching functions—I have yet to see a pediatric service designed with this in mind. Limiting the number of students per patient, enforcing rest periods and play periods, and strict observation of isolation procedures can help. An undocumented but obvious concern of too many visitors in a given ward is the danger of introducing infection. The unnecessary morbidity from hospital-acquired infection is surely aggravated by an increase in the number of individuals in close proximity to a patient. These problems should not be insurmountable when taken into consideration in designing a new hospital.

OPTIMAL HOSPITAL SIZE

A more difficult issue relates to the question of optimal hospital size. Most pediatric teaching programs function with seventy-five to 150 beds and clinics of varying size; children's hospitals tend to have from 150 to 600 beds, larger clinics, and busy emergency services.

The problems with being too small are obvious; bigness, on the other hand, can lead to an impersonal or "cold" environment. If service needs are met exclusively by resident physicians their numbers become excessive. When there are more than fifty interns and residents in pediatrics it is difficult for any one person to get to know them on an individual basis. Moreover house staff from family medicine programs on rotation in the clinics for two or three months may never have the opportunity to interact with the senior pediatric staff.

One approach to the question of "being too big" is to separate some of the service needs from the house staff rotations. I believe this approach is essential in a setting where the enterprise of the senior staff has brought to an institution relatively large numbers of certain kinds of patients who require many hours of staff time.

Neonatal intensive care units are one such example. If hundreds of very sick infants are brought to the hospital their needs are enormous and could consume a disproportionate share of house staff time. The recruitment of clinical fellows and an increase in full-time staff represent one solution; furthering the education and levels of responsibility of nurse specialists is another. Expanding the numbers of house staff, with the rationalization that they should meet all institutional service needs, may be incompatible with a balanced residency curriculum.

CONCLUSIONS

In conclusion, teaching and research are essential for the production of new ideas and new therapies. In the short term they keep children's hospitals competitive for patients who can find treatments there that are not available in an institution with no research capability of its own. In a very pragmatic sense, then, for the tertiary care institution to continue to attract patients, major support of research is needed. In the longer view, the achievements of preventive medicine should reduce the need to hospitalize children. Intensive care will probably always be needed for some, but care-by-parent and ambulatory care may make our present structures obsolete.

From a more general aspect, if university-affiliated children's services do not sponsor the kind of research needed to focus on some of the problems unique to children it is not likely that any other institution will do so. The sick child provides a continuing stimulus to investigators, who, in turn, promise to bring more immediate results from the laboratory to the bedside, and eventually to disease prevention.

THE ACADEMIC INTERFACE WITH DEPARTMENTS OF PEDIATRICS

THE ACADEMIC INTERFACE WITH DEPARTMENTS OF PEDIATRICS: OBSTETRICS AND GYNECOLOGY

Mortimer G. Rosen

INTRODUCTION

In preparing for this discussion I had some difficulty with the title assigned for my paper. On a practical basis I could understand the "charge," but the word "academic" disturbed me. As part of a university I know I am an academician; and as part of a community I know I am referred to as the "gown" in contrast to the "town" part of the scene. But what is an "academic interface"?

So quickly back to the books I went, and an older edition of the *Oxford Universal Dictionary*[1] referred me to Pluto and his academy. That truly was academic, but the association was a specific scholarly kind of education, and that really did not help me. In the same dictionary there was an allusion to academic skepticism (circa 1610), but this presented further difficulty as I did not want to speak about a skeptical interface with pediatrics. Continuing, I simplified my search by proceeding to the *Meriam-Webster Dictionary, Pocket Book Edition,* (large-type, easy-to-read version),[2] and chose as the definition for the term academic the *"theoretical rather than practical,"* and that is what I will speak about here: the theoretical rather than the practical interface between departments of obstetrics and gynecology and pediatrics. Obviously there are other meanings, but I will not belabor the point.

My reference materials for this theoretical talk include a
report of a conference sponsored in 1979 by the Josiah Macy,
Jr. Foundation, *The Current Status and Future of Academic Obstetrics,*[3] and a questionnaire I sent to sixty medical school department chairpersons in obstetrics. Finally I will discuss interfaces
between pediatricians and obstetricians in developed countries,
primarily those that take place in the United States.

BRIEF HISTORY

Let me first set the stage with a brief reference to the
historical evolution of departments of obstetrics and gynecology and then describe their present pediatric interfaces. Then,
as the data set upon which to speculate about where we may be
heading during the next ten years, I will use the responses to
the questionnaire from fifty-seven chairpersons and the medical practice setting at Cleveland Metropolitan General Hospital.

As the Bible tells us, obstetrics was present "in the beginning." While that initial birth reference suggests woman was
born of a rib of man, that is the last reference to male childbear-
ing I can find.

Early on, a woman's peers assisted in the birth process: for
the most part women helped women. In time these women
were replaced by specialists such as midwives. As men became
physicians and, ultimately, as manipulations to deliver im-
pacted babies were learned, and, later, as forceps were
introduced—albeit in secrecy—the delivery of the problem
pregnancy became the male physician's turf, and it remained
for men to deliver women.

During the late nineteenth and early twentieth centuries
pediatrics and obstetrics were closely linked. It appeared quite
satisfactory for the physician to deliver the mother and continue to care for the child. Specialists had not come into the
picture yet. The cesarean section was known, but it surely was
not used very often and for good reason—a parturient rarely
survived a cesarean birth. In the early 1900s it was reported to
be safer for a pregnant woman to be delivered following "gor-
ing" by a bull than in a New York City hospital by a surgeon.

One of our major journals of obstetrics and gynecology was

started in 1868 by a pediatrician, Abraham Jacobi. It was called *The American Journal of Obstetrics and Diseases of Women and Children;*[4] today it is known as the *American Journal of Obstetrics and Gynecology.*

In general, during this century specialty interests have grown rapidly and have culminated in a struggle for turf and in the creation of specialty boards. Pediatric care and obstetrical care separated bloodlessly. In the gynecological field, however, surgery performed on the female patient remained a battleground between the general surgeon and the obstetrician-gynecologist. Today this issue has been resolved in most large communities and in situations where both specialists exist in adequate numbers. In the absence of a gynecological surgeon, however, the general surgeon quickly assumes the technical aspects of this part of the specialty. In many residency programs there is still a mandatory surgical rotation. In certain schools, in order to be accepted for an oncological subspecialty training program, two years of general surgical training is preferred.

THE PRESENT

Again, for our understanding of today we must recognize the evolution of the medical practice or life-cycle pattern of the clinician. At the start of her/his years of clinical practice the graduate in obstetrics will primarily be visited by women as ambulatory patients, and this is soon followed by the growth of an obstetrical patient care load. Early in practice, gynecological surgery is minimal. Thus care of the pregnant woman is the way the clinician begins—and survives! With time, the patient load grows larger and more comfortable. The physician matures, and, despite the fact that today both small and large medical practice groups often replace the solo practitioner, the specialists in obstetrics-gynecology find that when possible they prefer not to work as many nights or on weekends.

This brings us to the middle years of a physician's clinical life span. By the late forties she/he is performing a great deal more gynecological surgery; the patients are the same women who delivered children fifteen years earlier. As this metamorphosis of clinical practice continues, gynecological surgery and office gynecology eventually predominate in the patient load. Finally the clinician relinquishes almost all the obstetrics in obstetrics and gynecology. I am sure there are many other reasons to explain this transition. Time will not allow further discussion, but the cycle of practice, the evolution of medical practice, is germane to my first major point.

Will Departments of Obstetrics and Gynecology Become Departments of Obstetrics and Pediatrics?

This question was not asked in the title of my talk, but it clearly must be addressed. It is important to note the pressures that were overcome to create the single discipline. Add to these the evolution of medical practice patterns discussed a moment ago and we find powerful forces working against this potential change. In my opinion neither the obstetrician nor the pediatrician will move easily into a combined discipline. Indeed, if anything, a growing practice called obstetrics and pediatrics as a specialty would only lead to more nights and weekends spent either in the hospital or on emergency call. And, as we know, that trend becomes harder for the individual to accept as she/he becomes older.

There are several examples of medical schools where combined departments of obstetrics and pediatrics functioned together without much evidence of success. Certainly, if the measure of the success of an idea is that others perceive it to be good and use it, this has not happened. Often these departments may meet pressure from their faculty and from their specialty boards. But whether or not the concept is good, the facts suggest that the idea of a combined department of obstetrics and pediatrics is not spreading to other medical schools. That gestation is at best described as growth-retarded.

As a further method of exploring subsets of the first question I constructed a questionnaire and sent it to sixty department heads (see the appendix to this chapter). The first question was:

Do you anticipate that obstetrics and gynecology will revert to two separate disciplines?

Fifty of fifty-five replies stated *no*. There seems to be no unanimity of thought, at least in this case. I did not ask specifically whether obstetrics and pediatrics will combine because I felt that question might arouse antagonism and thus color the responses. I asked that question more subtly, as we will see in later questions.

At my medical school, Case Western Reserve, I am unaware of any interest in much less pressure to combine the two departments. The individual administrative leaders are already so overwhelmed with their local and national obligations that to expand further is not a priority.

THE ACADEMIC INTERFACES
WITHIN THE SUBSPECIALTIES

There are, however, two areas, perinatal medicine and adolescent medicine, in which the academic departments clearly do overlap and the territoriality of the disciplines seems to become vague, or perhaps even to blend.

Here I must digress for a moment to look again at the outside forces that influence academic trends. The surge toward subspecialization first began in pediatrics with the creation of special care neonatal units. Neonatal intensive care units came to the forefront during the 1960s and reached a crescendo of change in the 1970s with the designation of tertiary, secondary, and primary care nurseries, infant transport programs, and special physicians to handle these special little people.

During the same years, perhaps as a response to this development in pediatrics, the movement began to flourish in obstetrics. Much earlier our obstetrical specialty recognized oncology and infertility as specialty areas, in fact if not by formal mandate. Obstetrics, or maternal and fetal medicine as it was soon to be called, lagged behind, perhaps because every obstetrician could deliver a baby: that training was basic. Or perhaps, as noted earlier, the generalist in obstetrics tended to move away from this aspect of the specialty, rather than toward it. Nonetheless maternal and fetal medicine was born, along with the subspecialties of oncology and endocrinology. Now let us discuss the interfaces between the pediatric subspecialty of neonatology and the obstetrical specialty of maternal and fetal medicine as they exist today.

MATERNAL AND FETAL MEDICINE AND NEONATOLOGY

Is there room for movement, or change, or evolution, or combination here? It is evident that the two subspecialty disciplines overlap in teaching and research, but it is of interest that they do not overlap as easily in patient care. First let us look at the next series of questions and answers from my obstetrical colleagues.

*Do you visualize a different specialty
orientation or amalgamation of neonatal
intensive care and maternal-fetal medicine?*

Yes: 19   *No:* 34

That suggests some motion, but follow the questionnaire more closely:

*Do you visualize a single specialist
for the two disciplines?*

Yes: 5   *No:* 49

Now we are back where we were with the initial question.

Collaboration: *Yes!*   Unification: *No!*

This is further buttressed by the next set of responses:

*Do neonatal specialists have joint
appointments in your department?*

Yes: 26   *No:* 29

*Is the reverse true—obstetricians
with appointments in pediatrics?*

Yes: 10   *No:* 44

We may speculate as to the meaning of these responses. There is a strong association and collaboration between these subspecialists, but the movement seems to be stronger from pediatrics toward obstetrics than in the reverse direction. Indeed at our hospital I have responded several times positively to requests for joint appointments; but no member of our maternal-fetal group has asked for a joint appointment in pediatrics.

Three other pieces of information are of interest:

Do your obstetrical residents resuscitate
neonates in the delivery room?
Yes: 46   No: 8
If no, do pediatricians resuscitate?
Yes: 26   No: 2
Do your obstetrical residents rotate
through the neonatal nurseries?
Yes: 45   No: 10
Do your pediatric residents rotate
through the obstetrical service?
Yes: 3   No: 52

What may we derive from these answers? Yes, obstetrical residents resuscitate neonates, but pediatric residents resuscitate them almost as often. It becomes clear that the barriers as to who "owns" the baby in the delivery room are breaking down—and that is for the good. If I extrapolate from these series of responses to our service at Cleveland Metropolitan General Hospital, what I see happening is this:

The first-year obstetrical resident always rotates through the neonatal intensive care nurseries for at least one month, often two. That is not voluntary; I believe it is extremely important for patient care, for understanding early newborn development, and for the establishment of good working relationships between residents in both disciplines.

In the unexpected delivery room emergency the obstetrician is well prepared to handle respiratory care, which, incidentally, is best taught in the neonatal intensive care unit. If a high-risk patient delivers or a cesarean is performed, however, the pediatrician is notified well in advance with, one hopes, the clinical case having been discussed in advance, and it is the pediatrician who waits to receive the baby and to administer respiratory care as needed.

On a rare occasion there is conflict. But, in general, during these moments of interface the obstetrician completes a technical procedure and prefers not to leave the mother. If obstetrical support is forthcoming it must be from other staff people. Thus continuity of care by a single person is almost, or often, impossible.

Add to this the response to the second part of the question: few pediatricians rotate through obstetrical services. One may speculate that this procedure may change, but my personal experience suggests it will not. I am not certain why this is so at our hospital, for we have opened up the program to pediatricians. Movement from pediatrics to obstetrics is not often seen. The family practitioner studies, and leaves the obstetrical service with skills to be used in practice; the pediatrician rarely enters.

The interfaces are less disparate in research and teaching. On the national scene more National Institutes of Health fetal study grants are awarded to departments of pediatrics[5] than to departments of obstetrics. Here continuity of study from fetus to neonate is maintained; research programs on problems of the low-birth-weight neonate and of the fetus are so closely aligned I believe this will persist.

At our hospital there is a great deal of overlap in research: more than forty active research protocols involve both obstetricians and pediatricians. We teach together and have overlapping consultations on patient care, on planning for the timing of maternal delivery, as in erythroblastosis, or on regulating maternal metabolism, as in diabetes.

But do I see a merger of the two into a single discipline? Not very likely. Single units of perinatal medicine have been set up as conjoined divisions in departments of obstetrics and departments of pediatrics. But I am unaware of any separation where responsibility for the mother, fetus, and infant has been taken out of the parent disciplines and merged into a single new category with departmental status. As may be seen from the answers to the questionnaire, this is not perceived as a probable evolution.

Now let us travel to the other end of the pediatric domain: What will happen in adolescent medicine?

ADOLESCENT MEDICINE

This area of special care is evolving as a response to a societal need and to a consequent shifting of priorities in both our specialties. Once again the concern arises first in departments of pediatrics, with obstetrics and gynecology, at this point, seemingly responding to pressure. In brief, some of the pressures leading to the formation of this discipline may be listed as:

Adolescent Gynecology as Seen by the Obstetrician:
- Sexuality
- Family planning
- Pregnancy and its many risks
- Venereal disease
- Gynecology

This list summarizes an obstetrician's view of this specialty area. The adolescent is a total person, however, and should be considered in a more complete context.

Adolescent Medicine as Seen by the Pediatrician:
- Physiological development
- Medical pathology
- Behavioral development
- Male and female persons

In this context there is far more to the person than the pelvis, or even the pelvis and its sexuality. The analogy exists between the internist and the obstetrician as the model that may evolve between pediatrician and obstetrician in the area of the adolescent. Clearly there is a pressing need for attention. The biological maturity of both males and females is evolving at an earlier age. And closely linked are the sexual activity patterns among adolescents. There is tremendous pressure on all of us to face these issues because in the United States 900,000 adolescent girls become pregnant annually, and some 330,000 have abortions. The rate of gonorrhea among adolescents age fifteen to nineteen is 1,212.4 per 100,000.[6] Thus the pressure for a new kind of physician is evident.

Let us look once again at the questionnaire:

Is there an adolescent medical program in your hospital?
Yes: 35   *No:* 19

Do you at any time admit obstetrical patients to pediatric hospital beds or to the adolescent floor?
Yes: 17   *No:* 38

Do pediatricians at your hospital give contraceptive information and care to adolescent patients?
Yes: 34   *No:* 21

It would appear that adolescent medicine is an emerging specialty in the discipline of pediatrics; the obstetrician, although delivering the babies of a large number of women in their adolescent years, remains only as a consultant. To meet this need adolescent obstetrical clinics are being formed. It is apparent that contraceptive education is essential in this age group. No longer is the young mother sent to a family planning clinic after delivery of her first baby. In our hospital, as is also evident from the questionnaire, the adolescent intrahospital service and the clinics dispense all forms of contraception. At first it was difficult to persuade pediatricians to assume responsibility for inserting the IUD. It was evident, however, that the person giving advice must feel comfortable in the use of all methods of counseling if that person was to be effective. And this evolution is occurring.

In Cleveland Metropolitan General Hospital antenatal and postpartum patients may be treated on the Adolescent Patient Floor. There are some problems connected with who takes the responsibility for that patient; but this too is changing. The pediatrician acts as the primary physician and the obstetrician as the consultant. The obstetrical resident makes daily rounds on the Adolescent Ward and interacts with the pediatric staff.

I see no movement by the pediatrician from the clinic or the inhospital patient to the delivery room. For this to occur the training programs will have to be altered, perhaps in a manner similar to those of family practice residents. With the increase in medical obstetrical risks among adolescents, however, and with the existing training programs and the attitudes and demands of the two different specialties I do not see this happening easily. And, once again, note the questionnaire: pediatricians are not receiving training in the delivery room.

In our hospital abortion patients are counseled, but they may not be admitted to the Adolescent Ward. This may be a result of resistance on the part of our nurses rather than of the pediatrician. As this is an adolescent problem I feel these patients should be bedded there when necessary.

Finally, gynecological patients are admitted to the Adolescent Ward and are managed by pediatricians in consultation with obstetrical residents. If the condition of the patient deteriorates—if, for example, the acute salpingitis becomes a pyosalpinx or pelvic abscess—then she is transferred to the gynecological service.

As a discrete subspecialty in the obstetrics-gynecology sphere there are certain conflicts I cannot resolve. Resident education, although woefully inadequate, must soon include adolescent medicine. As the program becomes stronger in pediatrics, residents will electively rotate through that service, perhaps during the second or third year of their program. Once the specialty is taught to the obstetrical resident, the obstetrical adolescent specialist will emerge. This person will appear first as the teacher, then as the clinician who specializes in adolescent gynecology.

Do I see this developing into a combined obstetrical-pediatric specialty instead of gynecology? Probably not, and for the same reasons discussed earlier.

Do I see adolescent obstetrics and gynecology becoming a subspecialty? Yes, I believe it will, in response to the demands of society, and because of its major societal costs; it will be taught in residency programs and then extended into clinical practice.

Do I see this evolving into a recognized, board-certified subspecialty? I am not sure. The first wave for establishing subspecialty boards has passed over us and has created many tides. Thirty percent of graduating obstetrical residents have stated they may take further subspecialty training.[7] At this time far less than 30 percent are entering fellowship programs. The national consensus, however—societal and governmental—is expressing some concern about specialty growth, and pressures are moving the neophyte physician toward medical practice as a generalist rather than as a specialist. That is why I am uncertain as to whether adolescent gynecology will evolve into a formal board-approved specialty: perhaps because of public opinion, or perhaps because that specialty would overlap the three basic specialties—endocrinology, maternal-fetal medicine, and to a lesser extent, oncology.

CONCLUSIONS

Let me try to summarize my discussion of the theoretical interfaces between our two specialties as I see them developing over the next decade:

• Obstetrics and gynecology is not likely to separate once again into two disciplines.

• Pediatrics and obstetrics are not likely to reunite into a single discipline.

• The field of perinatology can be expected to mature and expand in response to apparent needs. Interfaces will occur more often in patient care, education, and research. Perinatology is not likely to evolve as a single new specialty in the care of a single specialist.

• Adolescent medicine is a field more readily allied by its broad nature to pediatrics or medicine rather than to obstetrics. The subspecialty area of adolescent gynecology will grow within obstetrics and gynecology, but for obstetricians it will remain a consultative discipline, not a primary care discipline.

NOTES

1. W. Little, H. Fowler, and J. Coulson, *The Oxford Universal Dictionary on Historical Principles,* 3rd ed., rev. by C. T. Onims (Oxford: Clarendon Press, 1955).

2. H. B. Woolf, ed., *The Merriam-Webster Dictionary, Pocket Book Edition* (New York: Simon and Schuster Pocket Books, 1974).

3. J. Z. Bowers and E. F. Purcell, eds., *The Current Status and Future of Academic Obstetrics* (New York: Josiah Macy, Jr. Foundation, 1980).

4. F. H. Garrison, "History of Pediatrics," in I. A. Abt, *Abt-Garrison History of Pediatrics* (Philadelphia: W. B. Saunders, 1965): ch. I.

5. N. Kretchmer, "Support of Academic Obstetrics: The Public Sector," in *The Current Status and Future of Academic Obstetrics,* ed. J. Z. Bowers and E. F. Purcell (New York: Josiah Macy, Jr. Foundation, 1980): 42–57.

6. E. R. McAnarney, "Obstetrics and Pediatrics: Their Relationship in a Changing World," in ibid.: 153–60.

7. R. H. Messer, W. Pearse, and J. Fielden, "Academic Manpower for Obstetrics and Gynecology in the United States," *Obstetrics and Gynecology* 53, no. 5 (May 1979): 649–52.

APPENDIX

QUESTIONNAIRE SENT TO SIXTY HEADS OF DEPARTMENTS OF OBSTETRICS AND GYNECOLOGY IN THE UNITED STATES, 1980

ANALYSIS OF THE FIFTY-SEVEN REPLIES*

	Yes	No
1. Do you anticipate that the specialty of obstetrics and gynecology will revert to two separate disciplines?	5	50
2. Do you visualize our subspecialties aligning with other medical disciplines? For example:		
a) Oncological and gynecological surgery with pelvic surgery and general surgery?	10	45
b) Endocrinology and infertility with medical endocrinology?	6	47
3. a) Do you visualize a different specialty orientation or amalgamation of neonatal intensive care and maternal-fetal medicine?	19	34
b) Do you visualize a single specialist for the two disciplines?	5	49
c) Do neonatal specialists have joint appointments in your department?	26	29
d) Is the reverse true—obstetricians with appointments in pediatrics?	10	44
4. Do your obstetrical residents resuscitate neonates in the delivery room?	46	8
a) If no, do pediatricians resuscitate?	26	2
b) If no, do obstetricians resuscitate?	17	5

---

* Some replies in certain categories were incomplete.

APPENDIX (Continued)

5. Do your obstetrical residents rotate through your neonatal
   nurseries?*   45   10

6. Do your pediatric residents rotate through the obstetrical
   service?   3   52

7. Is there an adolescent medical program in your hospital? 35   19

   a) If so, what role does your department play in operating
      the program?†   —   —

   b) Does your hospital have an adolescent patient floor?†† 18   38

   c) Do you at any time admit obstetrical patients to pediatric
      hospital beds or to the adolescent patient floor?   17   38

8. Do pediatricians at your hospital give contraceptive information and care to adolescent patients?   34   21

		Increasing	*About the Same*	*Decreasing*
9.	Excluding oncology, is the level of gynecological surgical procedures at your hospital	24	15	16
10.	Are the number of oncological cases at your hospital	35	28	1
11.	Are the number of obstetrical admissions at your hospital	37	18	—
12.	Are the number of pediatric admissions at your hospital	18	21	12

* Four elective rotations are included in the yes category.

† The poor wording of this question did not allow for yes or no responses, so they have not been included here.

†† Four separate children's hospitals are included in the no category.

THE ACADEMIC INTERFACE WITH DEPARTMENTS OF PEDIATRICS: PSYCHIATRY

Leon Eisenberg

From the perspective of the pediatrician the title of a song from the musical *Pal Joey* epitomizes the academic interface with psychiatry: "Bewitched, Bothered, and Bewildered." Some few pediatricians have been bewitched by the magic promise of psychiatry and transmute pediatric visits into psychoanalytic investigations. Others are bothered by claims that leap ahead of evidence; by theories impervious to disproof by fact; and by psychiatric colleagues who refuse to share information on grounds of confidentiality. Most are simply bewildered by differences in work styles and by the difficulty of translating psychiatric recommendations into pediatric realities.

As viewed by psychiatrists, pediatricians are poorly prepared to deal with psychological issues because of inadequate training—a view echoed from within pediatrics itself;[1] they are sometimes dismissed as too zealous in the pursuit of esoteric diseases to be willing to listen to their patients; and occasionally they are put down with the odious remark that they resist psychodynamic interpretations because of their own unanalyzed psychopathology. For the pediatrician so labeled, trial is by a hanging jury. She/he has the pleasant options available to the defense at medieval trials of witchcraft: the accused is held below the surface of the water on the premise that drowning establishes innocence whereas survival proves guilt.

There is blame enough for all. Pediatricians are justly angry at psychiatrists, who claim to be doctors but who tell the family to call the pediatrician when a crisis arises at night. Psychiatrists may not be the only physicians with atrophic expository skills, but too many of us attempt to conceal our ignorance with a smoke screen of words. Yet pediatricians who are contemptuous of psychiatry because of its scientific limitations can ill afford to be uncharitable; medical diagnosis and treatment rest far more on a shaky base of belief and custom than pediatricians are ready to admit.[2,3] Pediatric house officers generally regard psychiatry as irrelevant, and too often they are reinforced in this attitude by their attendings. Let me also acknowledge that psychiatric residents tend to be uncomfortable with medical responsibility and to avoid experience on pediatric wards in favor of working within their own department where they feel safe.

Over the last two decades, battles over turf have heightened conflicts. Fewer children because of a declining birth rate, more family practitioners, and the greater ability of generalists to treat pediatric disorders because of medical progress have resulted in a more competitive marketplace. In consequence, pediatrics is elbowing psychiatry on the one side and neurology on the other in an effort to establish clinical hegemony over learning disorders, developmental disabilities, behavior problems, and the like.

This is reminiscent of the 1960s, when effective lobbying by parents' groups and the fortuitous circumstances of a president with a disabled member in his family resulted in the allocation of new resources to the field of mental retardation. In that decade pediatrics and psychiatry, both conspicuous for their longstanding neglect of the retarded, suddenly were born again in the struggle for control of a newly respectable domain. I do not fault the new interest in behavioral pediatrics, any more than the earlier conversion to mental retardation. Self-interest is quite reasonable as a motive for doing good. It may even be more enduring than spiritual salvation. What is to be avoided is hypocrisy.

Much more remains to be said about the mote in the psychiatric eye, but this is not the occasion for it. Let me instead limit my further remarks to the identification of the major barriers to the incorporation of psychosocial knowledge into pediatric practice, and to ways to overcome those barriers. As I see them, they are: the context of training; the constraints on practice; and the seductiveness of technology, whether behavioral or biological.

DECISIVENESS OF CONTEXT

Trying to teach psychological medicine to pediatric house staff is a discouraging experience. Medical students tell me I am a good teacher; my self-regard is further heightened by invitations to return to speak at pediatric postgraduate courses. Yet I recall many teaching conferences for pediatric residents at Johns Hopkins and at Harvard when my audience was a fraction of those who flocked to sessions on histiocytosis and sister chromatid exchange; when those who did come were glassy-eyed or falling asleep; and when they and I were equally dispirited by a leaden atmosphere I was unable to dispel.

One clue to my difficulty was provided by a young resident who may have been irregular in his attendance but certainly was consistent in his distaste. After his obligatory two years in the armed forces he returned to Hopkins for an alumni meeting. He sought me out to complain that he had received precious little in the way of psychiatric training. Yet in caring for military dependents he had been called on far more often for behavior problems, school difficulties, and marital discord than for the "interesting" diseases he had learned to manage so well at the Harriet Lane Home. What had seemed irrelevant had suddenly become vital.

The context of teaching provides an explanation for the paradox of my failure with the house staff and my success with practitioners. The fault lies with the discrepancy between what I try to teach and what matters to house officers. Their days and nights are occupied in caring for desperately ill, hospitalized children and in mastering the pathophysiology of disease on which the successful care of patients so crucially depends. The questions asked on rounds by pediatric attendings, who provide models of future professional behavior for the house officer, center on biological disease processes rather than on psychosocial pathology, unless the latter is so overwhelmingly intrusive as to be unavoidable.

Under such circumstances, to ask a house officer to learn about psychological development and its deviations is a bit like a demand to learn French when none of the patients seems to speak it. If a resident is prepared to listen at all, it can only be on the faith that the information will someday be useful or because pediatric boards demand it. She/he does not have to be urged to learn clinical pharmacology; it clearly matters to patient care and to one's own status in the training program.

I therefore conclude that *effective teaching of psychological pediatrics demands a context in which the house officer is responsible for providing continuous primary care to a substantial panel of ambulatory patients;* confronted by the demands of clinical reality, the resident will insist on learning what is now disdained as remote and irrelevant. The new residency training requirements of the American Board of Pediatrics will facilitate the attainment of this objective. I do not, however, plan to hold my breath until the requirements are fully implemented at academic medical centers.

FINANCIAL CONSTRAINTS ON PEDIATRIC PRACTICE

If the problems families bring with them make the practicing pediatrician more receptive to psychiatric instruction, the context of practice impedes the effective utilization of that information. Taking a psychosocial history, completing a thorough examination, discussing the implications of the findings, and providing continuous pediatric counseling all demand time. The process may not need a fifty-minute hour but it is just about impossible to do in a five- to seven-minute visit. Existing reimbursement schemes in fee-for-service medicine, had they been designed for the purpose, could hardly have been more effective in constraining the practice of psychologically informed pediatrics. Indeed the teaching hospital is not exempt: cost accounting and the managerial press to avoid deficits result in demands for "efficiency" in "processing" out-patients, all too often to the exclusion of the time needed for the neophyte to learn to explore psychosocial issues.

This audience does not need to be reminded that pediatricians are the lowest-paid specialists. Is it reasonable to expect even a conscientious pediatrician to lower his income further by seeing fewer patients in order to give those patients he sees additional time? If gastroenterologists have been transformed into endoscopists[4] and cardiologists into expert threaders of arterial catheters, should we be surprised to find pediatricians adroit at avoiding questions that may evoke lengthy answers so long as time is money? I therefore conclude that *the incorporation of psychological medicine into office practice demands a major change in the present fee system;*[5] the conscientious pediatrician who spends time educating and counseling patients should receive a fee appropriate to time well spent rather than be penalized by loss of income for providing what the patient needs. Without this change I am pessimistic that even the best psychiatric teacher and the most eager pediatric audience will be able to influence present modes of practice.

BEHAVIORAL MEDICINE: PROMISE AND PERIL

The 1970s have seen the emergence of "behavioral medicine," which is based on the application of learning theory to the management of behavioral problems and physiological disorders.[6] The tenets of behavioral medicine are more attractive to the practicing pediatrician than most psychiatric theories because they are simple, lead to specific therapeutic maneuvers, and yield tangible benefits in real time. Because ours is a pragmatic society we assume that what works is true. There is in fact a substantial gap between theory and practice in behavioral medicine.

Biofeedback has been "in" since a remarkable paper by Neal E. Miller in 1969;[7] he presented data that appeared to demonstrate the learning of visceral and glandular responses in rats that had been curarized to preclude voluntary muscle activity. Subsequent human studies demonstrated that heart rate, blood pressure, skin temperature, EEG rhythms, and muscle tension could be modified by conditioning. Unfortunately, as

Miller was the first to report, he and others have been unable to replicate the original animal experiments.[8] Moreover, most clinical investigators now find that simple relaxation methods yield as good, if not better, results than biofeedback in controlling blood pressure, headaches, and peripheral vasoconstriction.[9,10] With some important exceptions it now appears that costly biofeedback instrumentation is an unnecessarily complex way to teach patients how to modulate responses to stress.

I mention these developments not to discredit the importance of behavioral medicine, but to caution against confusing the appurtenances of science—instruments and laboratories—for the scientific method itself. Behavior therapies *are* a considerable advance in helping patients and their parents to manage problem behaviors, but they do not displace what remain as essential issues in the clinical encounter: the human meanings and the human values comprehensible only in the frame of the social and psychological theory. The peril in behavioral medicine is the substitution of gimmickry for a sensitive analysis of the life situation of the patient. Surely it will be helpful for the child with headaches or asthma if relaxation methods yield symptom relief. Yet a good doctor will not treat pain by analgesics without at the same time searching for causes; the same commitment requires that sources of tension within the family be explored and corrected where possible, rather than limiting action to the removal of the symptoms that are the manifest expression of stress.

Furthermore, it still remains to be demonstrated that the results of behavior therapies, though they are generally effective in the short run, can be sustained over longer time spans.[11] Problems in enhancing the generalization of new learning beyond the office encounter and in designing reinforcement schedules compatible with the patient's life environment remain to be solved.

PSYCHOLOGICAL PEDIATRICS AND THE PRACTICE OF MEDICINE

The ability to respond to a patient as a person, as well as to the disease that disables her/him, has always been the hallmark

of good clinical medicine. Regrettably, the very accomplishments of modern biomedicine in identifying and correcting disease pathophysiology has unwittingly distracted attention from the interpersonal issues that are inescapably a part of
the human experience of sickness. It has fallen to psychiatry to
be the standard-bearer for the thesis that medicine is a social as
well as a biological science.[12] It need not of course have required psychiatrists—not all are effective at teaching it; indeed
some, in striving for respect in biomedical circles, have become
indifferent to social context.[13] In pediatric departments with
superb clinicians this function of the psychiatrist is superfluous;
in all too many, only the psychiatrist serves as advocate for
comprehensive care.

In this connection it is useful to distinguish between disease
as conceptualized by physicians and illness as experienced by
patients.[14] Doctors diagnose and treat diseases, that is, abnormalities in the structure and function of body organs and systems. Patients suffer illnesses, that is, experiences of unwel-
come changes in state of being and in social function. Disease
and illness do not stand in a one-to-one relationship. Similar
degrees of organ pathology may generate quite different reports of pain and distress; illness may occur in the absence of
disease. Community surveys regularly identify many more persons who are symptomatic and many more who have abnormal
findings than are under medical care at any given time.[15]

Patienthood is a psychological rather than a biological
state; a person becomes a patient by consulting a physician.[16] It
is not that the presence or absence of disease is irrelevant,
either to the experience of illness or to the decision to see the
doctor, but that disease in itself is neither necessary nor
sufficient to account for the transition from personhood to
patienthood. In the presence of life stress, symptoms are more
likely to be experienced and are more likely to lead to a search
for help; indeed, as D. Mechanic has demonstrated, psychosocial stress proves to be as strong a predictor of the decision to
consult a doctor as is the presence of physical findings.[17] K. J.
Roghmann and R. J. Haggerty, in a study of a random sample
of 152 young families, asked each mother to keep a diary in
which she recorded daily the occurrence of upsetting events in

the family. Analysis of the data in relation to illness episodes and to the use of medical care revealed that stress in the family *increased* the utilization of care for the child when the child was ill, and *decreased* visits to the doctor for the mother herself when she was ill.[18]

In short, the physical abnormality found when a patient comes to the office does not necessarily provide a sufficient explanation of the reason for the consultation. The doctor who fails to inquire about family circumstances does not treat the patient adequately and may well encounter "noncompliance" because the prescription has not dealt with the underlying complaint. Thus the education of the pediatrician in psychosocial medicine is not a matter of preparation for the sub rosa practice of psychiatry; plainly and simply it is preparation to become an effective doctor.

THE PEDIATRICIAN AS "INFORMED CONSUMER"

I would distinguish severe psychiatric disorders from the psychological context of pediatric care and from the common behavior problems. It does not seem reasonable to expect most pediatricians to undertake to treat severely disturbed children, although the occasional pediatrician with special interest and special competence may well find this possible. The educational task is to make the pediatrician an "informed consumer" of available psychiatric information on diagnosis, management, and outcome. That is, the content of psychiatric education in pediatric training should enable the pediatrician to recognize such disorders; to know how to help families to select the best treatment from among the range of competing treatments in the marketplace; and to monitor the care the patient receives in order to be certain that it is of good quality. Pediatricians should become discriminating readers of the psychiatric literature without having to become experts in its details, just as they must know enough biostatistics and epidemiology to read the journals in their own field. Lectures, case presentations, videotapes, and selected readings are the appropriate educational modes for this aspect of training.

THE MORE THINGS CHANGE,
THE MORE THEY REMAIN THE SAME

I lay no claim to the discovery of the wheel. Much the same points were made some fifty years ago in an interchange between a pediatrician and a psychiatrist, both leaders in their day. Joseph Brennemann declared fervently that "the menace of psychiatry . . . is already seriously in our midst."[19] He castigated the overpopularization of child psychology, the improper use of psychological tests, and the dogmatic claims of psychiatric theorists. He warned against "bewildering nomenclature" and "confusion of theory and authority." What Brennemann so vigorously criticized was a menace *to* psychiatry rather than the menace *of* psychiatry.

James Plant responded to Brennemann's polemic with a paper entitled "The Promise of Psychiatry," addressing pediatricians in the following words:

> We are, as a people, going through great changes in the matter of human relationships. Whether you like it or not, the families which are your clientele are finding themselves face to face with new and profound social problems. . . . You cannot escape these problems and their implications to the child's health by deprecating them. . . . The promise of psychiatry is the promise that if the pediatrician will address himself to these problems he will face a vista of rare challenge. . . . Personally, I am sorry if he is only afraid of that challenge.[20]

In arguing for the incorporation of sound psychological principles in pediatric practice I do not pretend to have ready answers for all the problems pediatricians face in patient care. I insist only that such problems have always been, and will remain, part of medical practice. We serve our patients ill when we avoid the human quandaries manifest in illness behavior rather than grapple with them as best we can. In meeting that challenge, pediatrics will handicap itself if it does not assimilate what social science can contribute to the understanding and management of patient problems.[21-23]

NOTES

1. J. P. Shonkoff, P. H. Dworkin, A. Leviton, et al., "Primary Care Approaches to Developmental Disabilities," *Pediatrics* 64 (1979): 506–14

2. Harvard Child Health Project, *Children's Medical Care Needs and Treatments,* vol.II (Cambridge, Massachusetts: Ballinger Publishing Co., 1977).

3. L. M. Koran, "The Reliability of Clinical Methods, Data and Judgments," *New England Journal of Medicine* 293 (1975): 642–46; 695–701.

4. H. M. Spiro, "My Kingdom for a Camera—Some Comments on Medical Technology," *New England Journal of Medicine* 291 (1974): 1070–72.

5. Institute of Medicine, *A Manpower Policy for Primary Health Care* (Washington: National Academy of Sciences, 1978).

6. G. E. Schwartz and S. N. Weiss, "Yale Conference on Behavioral Medicine: A Proposed Definition and Statement of Goals," *Journal of Behavioral Medicine* 1 (1978): 3–12.

7. N. E. Miller, "Learning of Visceral and Glandular Responses," *Science* 163 (1969): 434–40.

8. N. E. Miller and B.R. Dworkin, "Visceral Learning," in *Cardiovascular Physiology,* ed. P. A. Obrist (Chicago, Illinois: Aldine, 1974).

9. K. Frumkin, J. R. Nathan, M. F. Prout, et al., "Nonpharmacological Control of Essential Hypertension in Man," *Psychosomatic Medicine* 40 (1978): 294–320.

10. E. T. Beaty and S. N. Haynes, "Behavioral Intervention with Muscle-Contraction Headache: A Review," *Psychosomatic Medicine* 41 (1979): 165–80.

11. A. J. Stunkard and S. B. Pennick, "Behavior Modification in the Treatment of Obesity: The Problem of Maintaining Weight Loss," *Archives of General Psychiatry* 36 (1979): 801–06.

12. L. J. Henderson, "The Practice of Medicine as Applied Sociology," *Transactions of the Association of American Physicians* 51 (1936): 8–22.

13. L. Eisenberg, "Interfaces between Medicine and Psychiatry," *Comprehensive Psychiatry* 20 (1979): 1–14.

14. ———, "Disease and Illness: Distinctions between Professional and Popular Ideas of Sickness." *Culture, Medicine and Psychiatry* 1 (1977): 9–23.

15. K. L. White, T. F. Williams, and B. G. Greenberg, "The Ecology of Medical Care," *New England Journal of Medicine* 265 (1961): 885–92.

16. L. Eisenberg, "What Makes Persons 'Patients' and Patients 'Well'?," *American Journal of Medicine* (in press).

17. D. Mechanic, "Effects of Psychological Distress on Perceptions of Physical Health and Use of Medical and Psychiatric Facilities," *Journal of Human Stress* 4 (1978): 26–32.

18. K. J. Roghmann and R. J. Haggerty, "Daily Stress, Illnesses and the Use of Health Services in Young Families," *Pediatric Research* 7 (1973): 520–26.

19. J. Brennemann, "The Menace of Psychiatry," *American Journal of Diseases of Children* 42 (1931): 376–402.

20. J. Plant, "The Promise of Psychiatry," *American Journal of Diseases of Children* 44 (1932): 1308–20.

21. M. B. Parloff, "Can Psychotherapy Research Guide the Policymaker?," *American Psychologist* 34 (1979): 296–306.

22. L. Luborsky, B. Singer, and R. Luborsky, "Comparative Studies of Psychotherapies," *Archives of General Psychiatry* 32 (1975): 995–1008.

23 L. Eisenberg and A. Kleinman, eds., *The Relevance of Social Science to Medicine* (Dordrecht, Holland: Reidel Publishing Co., forthcoming).

IMPACTS ON ACADEMIC PEDIATRICS

IMPACT ON ACADEMIC PEDIATRICS OF DEVELOPMENTAL PSYCHOLOGY*

Jerome Kagan

Theory and research on the child can aid both the scientific and clinical work of the pediatrician in three ways. First, scholarship on human development can provide explanations for clinical syndromes that have resisted understanding, and can refute or correct invalid or incomplete explanations; second, new data can provide the bases for more sensitive diagnostic procedures; and, finally, careful reflection on new empirical information can enhance our understanding of normal development and reduce parental uncertainties about aspects of their children's development.

This paper contains some examples of all three uses of developmental research. In order to communicate the remarkable progress made during the last twenty years I shall consider 1960 as the starting point and compare contemporary knowledge with the status of information two decades earlier.

NEW EXPLANATIONS

The Causes of Reading Disability

Difficulty in reading English prose is recognized as a frequent problem among American children; as many as 15 per-

* The preparation of this paper was supported in part by grant HD-10094 from the National Institute of Child Health and Human Development, and by National Science Foundation grant BNS78-24671, and National Institute of Mental Health grant 2T32 MH14581 04 to the Center for Advanced Study in the Behavioral Sciences.

cent of the children in selected cities are diagnosed as reading disabled.[1] This relatively high proportion is not replicated in all modern nations; on the Isle of Wight, for example, M. Rutter reported a rate of 4 percent, in contrast to 10 percent in England as a whole.[2] Estimates of the frequency of serious reading problems, however, may be inflated by investigators who equate reading disability with a relative difficulty in reading skills; if a child who reads at grade level, for example, happens to be in a classroom with many talented children who read above grade level, that child may be misdiagnosed as reading disabled.

Like most psychological phenomena, reading disability can be the product of relatively independent influences. Some potential sources of reading difficulty are inherited or acquired anomalies in central nervous system structure or function; defective vision or hearing; poor language skills; hostility toward the schoolteacher; or minimum motivation for school mastery. A child who reads below grade level invites analysis.

There is moderate consensus among educators, psychologists, and physicians that, within the large heterogeneous group called the reading disabled, there may exist a much smaller group who have adequate IQ scores; excellent vision and hearing; a mastery of English; a middle-class upbringing; no evidence of brain damage; and a positive attitude toward school. Despite these benevolent characteristics, these children read two or more years below their expected grade level. Some professionals call this small special group dyslexic. Although we, along with others, believe that dyslexia is not a particularly useful diagnostic label, that prejudice is unimportant. The need is to clarify the predisposing conditions for and attributes of the children with these special characteristics.

The popular hypothesis for many years was that dyslexic children did not perceive visual information accurately, especially letters in words. The major evidence for this idea was that reading disabled children often misread letters, especially visually confusable ones: they read *pot* for *dot* or *bad* for *dad*. This fact seemed to suggest that they saw a *d* as a *p* or as a *b*. Because these observers did not bother to administer a recognition test in which the child was asked to match letters or words, the hypothesis had a longer life than was necessary.

There is now a great deal of research indicating that the errors made by reading disabled children are least likely to involve reversals of letters, and that over 95 percent of reading disabled children perceive the letters correctly.[3] If the child is shown a triangular arrangement of words, with the word *dug* on top and the words *dug* and *bug* on the bottom, and is asked to match one of the words on the bottom with the word on top, most reading disabled children solve this problem with very few errors. The vast majority of reading disabled children who have normal vision do not have any perceptual disability in the visual mode.

This statement is also true for the auditory mode. My colleagues and I have been studying a group of thirty-five reading disabled Caucasian boys age eight to twelve, from intact, middle-class, monolingual homes, and their matched controls who are reading well. Not only do the reading disabled children perceive letters accurately, they perform well when asked to make exceedingly difficult auditory discriminations. For example, the reading disabled boys had no trouble discriminating *episcotister* from *etiscopister* or *eliskopel* from *elispokel*. This finding is in accord with similar work by S. Naidoo.[4]

Thus research has refuted the popular hypothesis that dyslexics have a perceptual deficiency. But, as K. R. Popper has noted, it is always easier to refute an incorrect explanation of a phenomenon than to discover a correct one.[5] Although we cannot replace the perceptual deficit explanation with a better etiological statement, there are signs of initial progress.

First, even relatively homogeneous reading disabled children who are not bilingual, have no obvious central nervous disorder, do not come from low-income backgrounds, and do not have low IQs (the traditional definition of dyslexia) display many different cognitive profiles of performance. After a careful study of 271 dyslexic boys, Naidoo concluded that

> the absence of clearly defined subgroups and the indications of a multiple rather than a unitary causation do not support the view that aetiologically or clinically separate forms of dyslexia can be distinguished.[6]

One provocative finding in our own work is that about one-third of the reading disabled group show unusually long reaction times in deciding on the validity of sentences such as "salt is white" or "plumbers print maps" administered over a two-year period. Briefly, the children were asked to decide, as quickly as possible, whether a particular orally presented sentence was true or false and to press a key to indicate their decision. The control children and about two-thirds of the reading disabled boys typically took between 500 and 700 msec. to decide on the validity of sets of sentences; but about one-third of the reading disabled boys had markedly longer mean decision times: about 700 to 900 msec. Three of the reading disabled boys had extremely long latencies; mean decision times of over 1 sec., and decision times for individual sentences of as long as 3 sec. Further, the correlations reflecting the intraindividual stability of mean decision times to varied sets of sentences ranged from 0.5 to 0.8.

Most important, the children who had long decision times to the orally administered sentences also had long decision times to pictures that were ecologically valid or invalid. For example, they were shown a picture of a purple carrot or a red apple and asked to decide its ecological validity. The fact that the children who had long decision times to the sentences also had long response times to the pictures suggests that this small group of reading disabled boys had difficulty in evaluating symbolic information.

Our tentative explanation of these data rests on the important finding that the boys with mean decision times greater than 800 msec. were capable of fast times on about one-third of the items. Unusually long decision times occurred with another one-third of the items, typically sentences containing less familiar words—trees are in the forest; lawyers defend couches. This profile suggests that among the children called dyslexic, no more than about one-third have a very specific cognitive deficit that makes it difficult for them to sustain the evaluative mental set necessary to extract the meaning of symbolic information and relate it to their knowledge automatically and efficiently.

The psychological functions that make it easy for most children to continue to have decision times of less than 700 msec. for twenty to thirty items may fail every minute or two in this small group of reading disabled children. As a result their decision times are prolonged on about one-third of the items.

This interpretation is supported by the fact that the decision times were longer for sentences at the end of the test procedure than they were for those at the beginning. Thus S.T. Orton's original theoretical suggestion that dyslexic children had a central nervous system lesion is likely to be correct,[7] but this diagnosis is probably appropriate for only a very small proportion of dyslexic children. Most important, the problem is not perceptual but profoundly cognitive.

Attachment and Its Measurement

Ever since the introduction and dissemination of conditioning and psychoanalytic theory after 1910, the concept of the infant's attachment to its mother became a topic of research and of heated discussion. Although nineteenth century observers were concerned with the mother's eventual bonding to her infant, they were relatively indifferent to the infant's attachment to the mother. In 1875 Elizabeth E. Evans asserted that "the strongest human tie is understandably that which binds a mother to her child."[8] But nowhere in her book, *The Abuse of Maternity,* did she say that the infant naturally bonded itself to the mother. Similarly, the child psychologist William Stern did not regard the infant's attachment to the mother as very strong:

> How quickly the little child gets used to a new nurse, even when it had great affection for her predecessor; how little the child misses—perhaps after short pain at parting—its parents when they leave home or a favorite animal.[9]

Many eminent contemporary theorists contend that the less diluted the relationship between caretaker and infant—the more we approach the relationship of one caretaker to one infant—the greater the likelihood of creating a special emotional disposition in the infant as a result of a secure attachment relationship.[10-12] A key supposition is that the more secure the infant's attachment to the mother, presumably based on minimal dilution of the interaction between infant and caretaker, the greater the child's ability will be to cope with future psychological stress. Future research might prove this idea to be valid, but it is important to note that, before the end of the first year, mothers in most societies share caretaking responsibilities with older daughters, and have done so for centuries. If this practice produced insecure infants and adults with fragile defenses one would expect these societies to have abandoned the practice. Since they have not, perhaps no natural law is being violated. In these contexts of course the children continue to have contact with the mother, or at least with the same caretaker. They are not being shifted from one set of caretakers to another, as occurs in repeated removals from foster homes in more modern nations. I suspect that the preoccupation with the infant's attachment to the mother, which increased dramatically after World War II, was due to a projection of adult anxiety onto the infant.

The major theoretical advance came when John Bowlby saw a way to synthesize ethological data, information on primate behavior, and psychoanalysis into the bold and apparently correct suggestion that the human infant, like other mammalian infants, develops a special relationship with its primary caretaker.[13] The work of other psychologists, especially that of M. D. S. Ainsworth[14] and L. A. Sroufe,[15] indicates that the attachment concept is theoretically useful. Its function seems to be to protect the young infant from distress and anxiety, for it is less likely to show behavioral signs of uncertainty—crying, inhibition of play, and clinging to the caretaker—to unexpected or unfamiliar events if it is in the presence of a target of attachment. Indeed the ability to buffer, prevent, or reduce uncertainty is at the core of the definition of attachment.

During the late 1950s Ainsworth suggested that separation anxiety—distress over the departure of the mother—and the reaction to the mother's return were sensitive indices of the infant's attachment.[16] The idea behind her laboratory assessment was that the eight- to twelve-month-old child who had developed a secure attachment to the mother should be distressed by her departure and should seek her upon her return. Infants who did not cry on the departure and who did not seek the mother upon her return were regarded as less securely attached. This concept made intuitive sense to many and seemed to fit empirical data, and as a result it became extremely popular. Indeed Ainsworth's "strange situation" procedure is now being implemented in laboratories around the world, and is the favorite index of the concept of secure/insecure attachment.

Recent research, however, has revealed that the tendency to cry following maternal departure shows similar developmental functions among children raised in a variety of settings:[17] at home or in day care centers in the United States; in *barrios* in urban Guatemala; in subsistence farming Indian villages in the Guatemalan highlands; in Israeli kibbutzim; and in !Kung San bands in the Kalahari desert; as well as among infants diagnosed as suffering from failure to thrive. Crying following maternal departure emerges at about age eight months, rises to a peak at thirteen to fifteen months, and then declines in all these groups. Moreover the developmental course of distress over maternal separation among blind children is not much different than that for children with sight.[18]

Because the growth function for separation anxiety is so similar in the foregoing settings, despite the fact that the amount of contact between mother and infant varies dramatically, it is likely that crying at maternal departure is due in part to the maturation of cognitive competencies. We have suggested that the principal competence is the enhancement of recall memory. Hence separation anxiety is not a sensitive index of the security of a child's attachment. Moreover the likelihood of seeking the mother when she reenters the room depends on how disturbed the child was when she left; if the child was not upset it is less likely to seek a reunion with the mother. Thus reunion behavior is confounded by the probability of the child displaying distress in the first place.

I believe that, at age ten months, after maternal departure the child generates from memory the schema of her former presence and holds that schema in active memory while comparing it with the present. If the child cannot resolve the inconsistency inherent in that comparison it becomes uncertain and may cry. One reason a familiar figure buffers the child's anxiety is because that person provides the child with opportunities for responses when uncertainty is generated. Recognition of the opportunity to initiate a familiar action toward a familiar person, or object, buffers uncertainty. Distress does not occur when the mother leaves the child with the father because the latter's presence provides the child with a potential target for its behaviors; that knowledge keeps uncertainty under control. Thus the reasons for separation anxiety and the ameliorative effects of the attachment figure on distress are profoundly cognitive.

In addition it is likely that temperamental factors make some contribution to the likelihood of displays of distress. R. B. Kearsley, and P. R. Zelazo, and I have shown that Chinese children, whether they are raised at home or in a day care center, are more likely than Caucasians to display separation distress.[19] Further, children who exhibit separation distress are more likely to show autonomic patterns suggestive of a vigilance set to visual and auditory information. And K. Tennes has demonstrated that in nonstressful situations children with high cortisol levels are more likely to become distressed after maternal departure than those with low cortisol levels.[20] This fact suggests the operation of a temperamental predisposition to distress in uncertain situations.

In sum, recent research has provided an important corrective to the initial hypothesis that the probability of distress and reunion behavior is a sensitive index of the security of an infant's attachment. It is now clear that cognitive maturity and temperamental disposition make substantial contributions to these phenomena. It may be that behavior in the separation situation reflects some aspects of the degree of security of the child's attachment to the caretaker. But the exact contribution of the child's relationship to the caretaker is still ambiguous. Once again empirical research has been of value in correcting a popular idea.

The Effect of Day Care on the Young Infant

Pediatricians are being asked with increasing regularity about the potential psychological consequences of day care for infants and young children. Ten years ago the popular view among psychologists, psychiatrists, and pediatricians was that day care during the first three years of life was probably pathognomonic. I believed this to be true, and spoke out against day care for infants on many occasions.

During the last decade, however, several major investigations of the effects of day care have been implemented. They indicate that if the ratio of caretaker to infants is not greater than 1:3 or 1:4, and if the infants have freedom to explore their environment and encounter tameable variety, their cognitive, affective, and social development are not obviously different from children being raised at home. This was the major conclusion our group reached in our own longitudinal study of the effect of day care on infants.[21] We found that Chinese and Caucasian children age three and a half to twenty-nine months who attended a day care center were not obviously different in their psychological characteristics than a matched group of children raised at home. Henry Ricciuti came to the same conclusion after his independent review of the literature on infant day care:

> On the basis of the research data available thus far, there appears to be no evidence to support the view that extended day care experience beginning in the first two years of life has a disruptive influence on the affectual relationships between infant and mother. In fact there are some data suggesting that under favorable circumstances such experiences may make it somewhat easier for children to adapt comfortably to unfamiliar social situations requiring a willingness to tolerate some distancing from mother. . . . There appears to be little or no persuasive empirical research evidence thus far indicating that infant day care experience is likely to have unfavorable developmental consequences. This is a valid generalization whether one considers the child's intellectual development, affectional relationships between child and mother or subsequent peer relationships and responsiveness to adult socialization influences.[22]

Even young children in institutional settings who are nurtured by many caretakers, and who are therefore exposed to discontinuity in the infant-caretaker relationship, can develop normative IQ scores.[23] This finding led Rutter to conclude that, "Continuities in family relationships do not have the central role in intellectual development that they do in social development."[24]

If each caretaker has too many infants to nurture and if they are not permitted to explore their environment or encounter variety they will of course show definite signs of serious cognitive retardation. The form of surrogate care does indeed make a difference; but group care per se does not seem to have obvious hidden dangers.

Research on the three issues described so far—the etiology of dyslexia, the meaning of separation anxiety, and the consequences of day care—have produced data that refute popular hypotheses. There are of course many other examples of the utility of recent developmental research. Twenty years ago most psychiatrists believed that autism could be produced by an overly harsh and rejecting mother; few believe that hypothesis today.[25] Many pediatricians and psychologists were sure a child's future IQ could be predicted by its functioning during the neonatal period; that hypothesis, too, has been refuted.[26] Furthermore, many people used to believe that irritability in a one-year-old was solely the product of the mother's handling technique; today we recognize that the infant's temperament contributes to its irritability. Two decades ago it was believed that most of the sex differences in behavior in American children were learned; today we appreciate that some differences are biological, for there seems to be a biological basis for sex differences in vigorous and aggressive play during early childhood. These advances in knowledge in a relatively short time indicate that, even in a relatively immature science such as developmental psychology, persistent and intelligent inquiry is useful.

DIAGNOSTIC PROCEDURES FOR
ABERRANT DEVELOPMENT

The physician does not yet have the diagnostic tools needed to make sensitive and valid assessments of psychological competencies, attitudes, motives, and mood states appropriate to different stages of development. Even if the physician has an hour to observe a child's dominant attitudes, moods, and motives, few reliable methods are available to permit assessments to be made.

A great deal of progress has been made in the assessment of cognitive functions and this has produced a new view among developmental psychologists. This new concept argues that it is not theoretically useful to regard cognitive development as consisting of a unitary competence that generalizes across all domains. Rather, it is becoming clear that we should regard cognition as composed of a set of specific mental abilities implemented in specific contexts with specific materials. Thus we should speak of "perceptual inference with social events" or "perceptual analysis of visual scenes," rather than of *perceptual ability*. We should talk about "recognition memory for words" or "recall memory for faces" rather than about *memory* in general. Each of these specific cognitive functions grows at different rates during different developmental periods. A diagnostic term applied to a child without a statement of the context is incomplete.

During the first two years of life, for example, there is little correlation between a child's level of language competence and its ability on nonlinguistic tasks, such as recall memory for locations, inferences regarding relative size, and maturity of symbolic play. In three separate studies with middle- and working-class Caucasian children we found these kinds of variables to be independent of each other.[27] Many investigators find correlations of less than 0.2 among recall memory performance for pictures, words, sentences, and numbers.

This lack of generality is not restricted to American or European children. M. J. Sellers found low correlations across a variety of memory tasks in rural Costa Rican children.[28] Similarly, B. Rogoff found low correlations between recall scores for orally presented sentences and visual scenes in preadolescent children living in northwest Guatemala.[29] Even among reading disabled boys there is no correlation between memory for words and memory for pictures, and no relation between recognition and recall memory. These results and conclusions are a far cry from suppositions that led to general constructs such as intelligence. The pediatrician should not conceptualize the child's mental ability in terms of a single construct such as the intelligence quotient, but should be concerned with assessing the child's recall memory for words, perceptual analysis of pictures, or inferences regarding human motivations. Let me illustrate this idea.

There appears to be a maturational enhancement of retrieval memory for concrete events in all infants between age eight and twelve months.[30] The seven-month-old child cannot remember where a small toy is hidden if there is a five-second delay between the time of the hiding and the child's opportunity to reach for the toy; the one-year-old solves that problem easily. The pediatrician who is worried about the integrity of the central nervous system in a one-year-old might take a few minutes to administer this diagnostic procedure: if, with a delay of five seconds, a one-year-old cannot remember where a toy is hidden, something is probably amiss in the child's development. Similarly, an eight-year-old should be able to remember five numbers, pictures, or words read in a sequence—for example, shoe, hair, lamp, car, banana; if the child can remember only three of these items there is reason to hypothesize anomalous development. John H. Flavell has shown that, after age seven, children use spontaneous strategies to aid their ability to remember unrelated material.[31] If they do not use these strategies a hypothesis of delayed cognitive development is reasonable.

Another important cognitive function is called evaluation. After age six children begin to realize that when an intellectual problem is difficult to solve it is adaptive to pause and examine all alternatives before responding; it is maladaptive to offer the first hypothesis without sufficient reflection on the validity of all alternatives. Japanese children develop a reflective tendency by age five or six; American children do so by age six or seven.[32]

Our group has developed a widely used test called the Matching Familiar Figures Test, in which a child is shown one picture of a meaningful object and six very similar pictures, only one of which is a replica of the standard; the child must select the replica from the six alternatives. This test can be administered by a pediatrician in about fifteen minutes. If a nine-year-old shows a mean reaction time of less than eight seconds and makes ten or more errors on the twelve-item test, that child is likely to be impulsive in contexts in which its intellectual ability is being assessed and may be having problems in school.

An important method developed over the last twenty years to assess a child's possession of concepts is called proactive interference. In this procedure a child is read three words belonging to a common category, let us say animals (dog, mouse, and giraffe, for example), and is then required to count backwards from 100 for about fifteen seconds to prevent rehearsal of those three words. At the end of fifteen seconds the child is asked to recall the three words. He is then given a second set of three different animal words, required to count back from 100, and asked to recall the three words. Finally, he is given a third trio of animals, is asked to count, and then to recall the words. Typically, most children can remember all three animal words in the first trio, about two in the second set, but none or perhaps one of the third.

Psychologists say there is interference in the recall of the third trio because the child automatically refers the animal words to a category. When that category is changed, for example, if the child is now given three words representing articles of clothing, he remembers all three. The deterioration in recall of the animal words across the three sets is evidence that the child is thinking conceptually. A ten-year-old should show proactive interference for common categories such as animals, foods, and clothing. If a child does not do so he might not be relating the symbolic information to a conceptual category; that is an important fact about his cognitive functioning.

J. Piaget's work also lends itself to office testing. He has shown that by age seven most children in civilized communities are at a stage of concrete operations. As a result they believe in a set of logical rules, such as transitivity and the conservation of substance. If a nine-year-old cannot conserve numbers or mass, that fact is evidence that should be pursued because of the possibility of a retardation in an aspect of cognitive development.[33]

Assessment of Attitudes

Although diagnostic procedures for evaluating a child's attitudes are far less powerful than the procedures for evaluating cognitive functioning, some new inventions show initial promise of being useful. Let us suppose a pediatrician wants to know how a child views its parents. Children are defensive about discussing such intimate topics in an interview, but some procedures slip by the child's censor. In one procedure a list of twelve to eighteen adjectives are utilized that describe certain psychological qualities such as kindness, affection, justice, type of punishment, and proneness to anger. The doctor names three people the child knows and asks him to indicate which two of the three are most alike for each of the psychological properties. For example, of the father, mother, and teacher, the child is asked which two are most similar in *kindness*. A similar question is asked for the other psychological traits. Examination of the child's answers reveals how the child views each parent. If the child eliminated the father from the trio for all nurturant dispositions, and eliminated the mother for all aggressive or harsh dispositions, it is likely the child perceives the father as less nurturant than the mother, although he might be reluctant to say so in an interview.

This technique is also useful in determining how a child perceives himself in the classroom; it is especially useful in determining if the child sees himself as an isolate or as similar to desirable or undesirable peers. To implement this technique the examiner needs the names of all children of the same sex in the child's classroom, typically ten to fifteen, and information from the teacher on how well the children are doing and how popular and dominant they are with others. The examiner constructs about three dozen triads from this group of peers, some of which include the child. He then names trios of children and asks the child to decide which two are most alike in their behavior. The resulting set of answers permits the examiner to determine if the child places himself with no other children, that is, sees himself as isolated, or with children who have either desirable or undesirable characteristics.

Recently in our laboratory thirty-five girls and thirty-five boys from four different public school classrooms in Cambridge were studied. Each child first ranked him or herself and all of his/her same sex peers in the classroom on five psychological attributes: academic skill; popularity; physical attractiveness; dominance with peers; and athletic skill. In addition, each child was given a set of triad judgments to make: he/she had to decide which two children in each of the triads acted most similarly. The children who were evaluated by their peers as being popular, dominant, and achieving generally evaluated themselves positively on those attributes. But the majority of the children who were ranked by most of their peers, and the teacher, as having undesirable qualities—poor reader, unpopular, easily dominated—did not acknowledge that fact in their own self-ranking or when asked directly. The triad procedure proved useful, however. For example, six children who ranked themselves as competent readers, but who were in fact very poor readers, aligned themselves with the poor readers in the triad procedure. Five children who were minimally dominant, but who denied this quality on the direct ranking question, placed themselves with the low dominant children in the triad.

The triad data added important information on attitudes about self for three-quarters of the children who had extremely undesirable characteristics. If investigators who asked children directly about their qualities had also used the triad procedure the likelihood of a more correct classification of a child with undesirable qualities might have been improved by about 75 percent.[34]

UNDERSTANDING DEVELOPMENT

Research on development provides a more complete understanding of ontogeny, and, by enhancing parents' knowledge, buffers their uncertainties.

The Preservation of Psychological Properties

Of great interest to parents and professionals is the question of what structures and functions are preserved in ontogeny, either in the same form, which is rare, or in altered form. For example, if it is true that an infant's attachment to the mother is necessary for later intimacy in adulthood, one would say that some psychological structure created in the first year was preserved, albeit in altered form.

Twenty years ago a great deal of the empirical research on early development was under the influence of two ideologies: psychoanalytical theory and intelligence testing. Both ideologies ascribed general qualities to the young child, assuming he possessed an internal disposition that was preserved, but that took different disguises during different periods of ontogeny. The child's intelligence was reflected in babbling to an examiner at four months; knowing the meaning of *orange* at age three years; and remembering five numbers at age six. Anxiety was indexed by feeding problems at twelve months; phobias at age four; and depression in early adulthood.

These were bold hypotheses, Platonic in conception, that captured the imagination of many scientists, myself included. Some of us went off like Don Quixote, attempting to affirm their obvious validity. I spent twenty years trying to generate quantitative proof that the differences in behavior seen during the first two years of life were preserved in some way for the next decade. The results of longitudinal studies, however, have failed to find support for the notion that the individual variation seen at age two in the vast majority of family-reared children is preserved for the next ten years.

We recently reviewed most of the evidence for the prediction of variation in psychological profile during late childhood or adolescence from variation in infant behavior.[35] The existing data do not lend strong support to the view that salient psychological characteristics of a two-year-old, created by variations in early handling as modified by infant temperament, are related in an obvious way to dispositions a decade later when social class is controlled.[36] Precocity in attaining the milestones of infancy is not predictive of higher IQ scores or higher levels of intellectual functioning in adolescents as long as the continuing effects of social class are controlled.[37] When the investigator does not remove, statistically or theoretically, the continuous influence of being reared in a particular ethnic or class setting, one typically finds modest relationships between variation in behaviors at age two and variation a decade later, especially for cognitive variables.

Young children from lower-class families who, for a variety of reasons, are late in attaining developmental milestones tend to attain lower scores on assessments of intellectual competence, typically IQ tests, during later childhood. But these children had spent all the intervening years in that environment; had they been exposed to an environment that promoted cognitive development between the ages of two and ten it is possible their talents might have been enhanced. Despite correlations approaching 0.4 between scores on the Gesell scale administered at nine and twenty-four months, M. Sigman and A. H. Parmelee noted:

> We are not too optimistic about predictions from the first year of life to the fifth year which do not incorporate the ongoing events and experiences within the child's life. . . . Predictions which do not take into account the ongoing transitions between child and environment are bound to be weak.[38]

The study of the stability of variation in noncognitive qualities during infancy, such as dependency on or irritability with the mother, also reveals little predictive relation to theoretically reasonable derivatives a decade later. The occurrence of problems during very early childhood, presumably due to family experience, is not related in any obvious way to symptoms in adolescence or adulthood.[39] Thus, even though the behaviors of parents influence a young child, often dramatically, and even though the child's profile at one year might predict his behavior six, twelve, or eighteen months later, it has been difficult to demonstrate that most of the child's early attributes have an indefinite life. It appears that some problems observed during the first two years continue for two or three more years and then gradually vanish, due, we suppose, to the therapeutic effect of new experiences. Indeed H. F. Harlow and his colleagues have demonstrated that even the stark consequences of rearing macaque monkeys in isolation can be altered.[40]

It is not that parental behaviors do not influence the young child; they do. But future experiences can be equally effective. Coherent patterns of dispositions or their derivatives persist, we believe, only when they remain adaptive. Since there is so much change in environmental demands during the early years, it is not surprising that psychologists have been unable to trace the profile of the ten-year-old to the experiences of infancy.

Clinical studies also fail to verify the necessary preservation of pathognomonic signs. After the Second World War the International Social Service arranged for middle-class American families to adopt homeless children, most of them from

Greece and Korea, who had lived uncertain lives during the war. When they arrived in the United States their ages ranged from about five months to ten years. Thirty-eight of these children were followed by a team led by Samuel Waldfogel of the Judge Baker Guidance Center in Boston. About eight of the thirty-eight were judged initially as displaying very severe signs of anxiety. The initial problems in the new adoptive homes were overeating, sleep disturbance, nightmares, and excessive clinging to the new parents. Over the years these symptoms vanished, and most of the children made good progress in school and showed no learning disabilities. The investigators concluded that:

> The degree of recovery observed in most cases could not have been predicted from the writings of those who have studied the effects of separation most carefully. The present results—tentative as they are— indicate that for the child suffering extreme loss the chances for recovery are far better than had been previously expected.[41]

Similar findings have come from studies by M. Winick[42] and by W. Dennis.[43]

Although the effect of the lack of a strong form of continuity from infancy to later childhood has still not been confirmed beyond doubt, the burden of proof has shifted from those who deny strong continuity to those who claim it exists. What does seem clear is that the child does not carry a quality through development that is independent of the context in which it lives. If future investigators demonstrate the preservation of some characteristics from infancy to adolescence it is likely to occur under conditions where the environment has promoted or has maintained the young child's particular psychological properties. For example, some four-month-old babies babble a lot; others are relatively quiet. This variation seems to be based in part on biological differences among children. A babbling infant born to well-educated parents will, two years later, be more talkative than a quiet four-month-old born to parents of the same social standing. But a highly vocal four-month-old born to less well-educated parents who do not encourage early vocalization will be no more talkative than a low-vocal middle-class infant. Infant qualities are not permanent attributes; they are continually subject to environmental pressures.[44]

After a careful review of the relevant literature Rutter concluded:

> We have come a long way from the early views that infantile experiences somehow fix personality and that therefore it was too late to remedy the faults of omission or commission in those vital pre-school years. However, it is evident that we have a long way yet to go before we can adequately appraise the long-term effects of early experiences. It is good that human resilience has proved to be greater than once thought. Continuities between infancy and maturity undoubtedly exist, but the residual effects of early experiences on adult behavior tend to be quite slight because of both the maturational changes that take place during middle and later childhood, and also the effects of beneficial and adverse experiences during all the years after infancy. While it is clear that the long-term effects of early deprivation depend heavily on whether or not the deprivation continues, it would be premature to conclude that infantile experiences are of no importance in their own right. That remains a matter still worthy of further study and one in which there is a surprising paucity of information.[45]

The crudity of modern psychological methods permits any reasonable person to maintain the traditional hypothesis of the stability of early characteristics. One should at least accommodate to the existing empirical information, however, and entertain the remote possibility that the profiles sculptured within the family during the first two years are not necessarily permanent, although some may persist if the context that produced them does not change. I suspect that the fragility of the behavioral profile seen during the first two years, in contrast to the moderate and acknowledged stability found after ages four or five, is due to the fact that the executive function we call self does not emerge until late in the second year. When that complex psychological process surfaces it turns the flux of experience into expectations that show some resistance to change.

As long as we conceptualize the contents of the mind as a pattern of iron filings we will be tempted to regard psychological structures as hardened steel rather than warm wax. Existing data are so fragile it is not possible to decide the issue of preservation of early properties solely on empirical grounds. So we ask: Is it logically possible that any set of structures or behaviors in a two-year-old might not be capable of alteration through application of proper experience at the proper time?

The data from existing studies do not provide much basis

for enthusiasm among those who contend that the experiences of the first two years create structures and action profiles that are relatively fixed and persist no matter what environmental circumstances follow. It is true that the existing corpus of data does not permit one to conclude that the experiences of infancy are of no consequence for later childhood. But the data do imply that, if the structures created by those early encounters are not supported by the child's current environment, one should be prepared to see dramatic changes.[46,47]

All this information is relatively recent and has not yet penetrated public consciousness. There is resistance to its implications because the reasons for maintaining faith in the primacy of early encounters are intuitively attractive. A particular recipe of interactions is still seen as an elixir young children need in order to obtain society's highly valued prizes. From John Locke through Bowlby there has been consensus that early experiences set permanent directions because everyone hoped that parents could control the future of and prevent anomalous development in their children. As the range and the mystery of variation in adult status has expanded from the eighteenth century to the present, the danger of being left out made parents seek some explanation for that variation. The suggestion that early experience was the primary force was partially satisfying because it resolved uncertainty; provided rituals that reduced parental anxiety; made material encounters between the child and his environment the bases for negative outcomes; and, above all, it was rational.

A Changed Conception

We are at the present time witness to an important change in the presuppositions that underlie developmental research. Two decades ago the dominant view among psychologists was that environmental experiences were the primary causes of the appearance, rate of growth, and individual variation of basic competencies. Separation anxiety, the first sentences, and self-consciousness, for example, were regarded as dependent on specific interactions children had with adults and objects. There is a growing appreciation, however, that during the early years of life the appearance of these and other basic properties of our species depends on maturation of the central nervous system. Just as we expect the child to stand at twelve months and walk at fifteen months, so, too, we expect an enhancement of memory at ten months; the appearance of the capacity for symbolism by thirteen months; awareness of standards by eighteen months; self-consciousness by twenty-three months; and the first sentences by twenty-five months. The principal role of the environment is in determining the velocity with which these dispositions develop.

In addition, we recognize that environmental experience interacts with the child's temperament in producing psychological surfaces. Sigmund Freud insisted that the child's constitution determined his vulnerability to neurosis; specific family experience determined the symptoms that would develop. But that insight was lost after 1920 when conditioning theory became widely accepted and material interactive experience between parents and children became the primary mechanism of psychological growth. We are returning in part to the view held by nineteenth century scholars: a given experience does not have the same effect on all children; all animals in a niche do not react similarly to an increase in lichens in the immediate environment. Parents should appreciate that although their actions with a child are influential, often extremely so, each child makes a contribution to its own development.

Contemporary theory in child development makes the mother-infant bond the central experience in the young child's life; this was not true several centuries ago. Historical study reveals that a profound change occurred in Europe during the early seventeenth century. The educated citizen of the fourteenth and fifteenth centuries apparently did not award the mother-infant relationship the same potency we do. Michel E. Montaigne believed that mothers were capricious, and attributed his adult character and personality to luck and to a father who was a good role model. Like other sixteenth century scholars he dismissed the formative influence of his own and other people's mothers. But by the mid-seventeenth century a woman's dignity and influence were being celebrated by middle-class Europeans. From Locke, Jean Jacques Rousseau, and

Thomas Jefferson through Freud, Bowlby, and Erik H. Erikson there has been a steady movement to make the mother the central factor in the child's development. Although future research may affirm this concept, even the most traditional scholar in child development would admit that it still remains largely unproven.

We must therefore explain why there is such strong emotion surrounding discussions of surrogate care for children, and what I believe is relatively uncritical acceptance of evidence indicating that an unbroken infant-mother relation in the first year is critical for the child's future development. A combination of emotional conviction and frail evidence often betrays the fact that a deep value is being threatened. In the present case I believe the possibility that the biological mother might be partially replaced bothers a great many citizens. Every society needs some transcendental themes to which it can be loyal. In the past, God, the beauty and utility of knowledge, and faithful romantic love were among the sacred ideas viewed as both beautiful and beneficial. Unfortunately the facts of modern life have made it difficult for many adults to be loyal to these moral propositions. The sanctity of the mother-infant bond may be one of the few transcendental ideas in modern America ideology that remains unsullied. The number of books and articles on the importance of mother-infant contact during the early hours and days of life seems to be generated by strong emotion, suggesting that something more than a scientific fact is monitoring the discussion. If the infant can be raised by any concerned adult, one more sacred column will have fallen.

The major function of research in the social sciences is to evaluate the validity of a society's folk theories. The true status of many unpopular beliefs regarding the influence of family experience on the child is still unclear; some may prove to be correct, others not. Until relevant information is gathered, the community must be patient and tolerate the ambiguity inherent in available knowledge.

NOTES

1. P. Satz, H. G. Taylor, J. Friel, et al., "Some Developmental and Predictive Precursors of Reading Disabilities: A Six-Year Follow Up," in *Dyslexia: An Appraisal of*

Current Knowledge, ed. A. L. Benton and D. Pearl (New York: Oxford University Press, 1978): 313–48.

2. M. Rutter, "Prevalence and Types of Dyslexia," in ibid.: 3–28.

3. F. R. Vellutino, "Toward an Understanding of Dyslexia," in ibid.: 61–112.

4. S. Naidoo, *Specific Dyslexia* (London: Pitman, 1972).

5. K. R. Popper, *Conjectures and Refutations* (London: Routledge and Kegan Paul, 1963).

6. Naidoo, *Specific Dyslexia* (See note 4): 109.

7. S. T. Orton, "Specific Reading Disability—Strephosymbolia," *Journal of the American Medical Association* 90 (1928): 1095–99.

8. E. E. Evans, *The Abuse of Maternity* (Philadelphia: Lippincott, 1875): 7.

9. W. Stern, *Psychology of Early Childhood up to the Sixth Year of Age,* 6th German ed. (New York: Holt, Rinehart, 1930): 531.

10. M. D. S. Ainsworth and S. M. Bell, "Attachment, Exploration and Separation Illustrated by the Behavior of One-Year-Olds in a Strange Situation," *Child Development* 41 (1970): 49–67.

11. J. Bowlby, *Attachment and Loss,* vol. 1 (New York: Basic Books, 1969).

12. E. H. Erikson, *Childhood and Society,* 2nd ed. (New York: Norton, 1963).

13. Bowlby, *Attachment and Loss* (See note 11).

14. Ainsworth and Bell, "Attachment, Exploration" (See note 10).

15. L. A. Sroufe and E. Waters, "Attachment as an Organizational Construct," *Child Development* 48 (1977): 1184–99.

16. Ainsworth and Bell, "Attachment, Exploration" (See note 10).

17. J. Kagan, R. B. Kearsley, and P. R. Zelazo, *Infancy: Its Place in Human Development* (Cambridge: Harvard University Press, 1978).

18. S. Fraiberg, "The Development of Human Attachments in Infants Blind from Birth," *Merrill Palmer Quarterly* 21 (1975): 315–34.

19. Kagan, Kearsley, and Zelazo, *Infancy: Its Place* (See note 17).

20. K. Tennes and J. W. Mason, "Developmental Psychoendocrinology," in *Measuring Emotions in Infants and Children,* ed. C. E. Izard (New York: Oxford University Press, forthcoming).

21. Kagan, Kearsley, and Zelazo, *Infancy: Its Place* (See note 17).

22. H. N. Ricciuti, "Effects of Infant Day Care Experience on Behavior and Development," unpublished manuscript (Ithaca: Cornell University, 1976): 34, 35, 40.

23. B. Tizard and J. Rees, "The Comparison of the Effects of Adoption, Restoration to the Natural Mother, and Continued Institutionalization on the Cognitive Development of 4-Year-Old Children," *Child Development* 45 (1974): 92–99.

24. M. Rutter, "The Long-Term Effects of Early Experience," Mary Elaine Meyer O'Neil Lecture, 1980.

25. ———, "Autism: Psychopathological Mechanisms and Therapeutic Approaches," in *Cognitive Growth and Development,* ed. M. Bortner (New York: Brunner Mazel, 1979): 273–99.

26. R. K. Yang, "Early Infant Assessment," in *Handbook of Infant Development,* ed. J. D. Osofsky (New York: John Wiley, 1979): 165–84.

27. J. Kagan, *Psychological Development in the Second Year* (Cambridge: Harvard University Press, forthcoming).

28. M. J. Sellers, "A Study of Memory" (Ph.D. diss., Harvard University, 1978).

29. B. Rogoff, "Memory Development" (Ph.D. diss., Harvard University, 1977).

30. Kagan, Kearsely, and Zelazo, *Infancy: Its Place* (See note 17).

31. J. H. Flavell and H. M. Wellman, "Metamemory," in *Perspectives on the Develop-*

ment of Memory and Cognition, ed. R. V. Kail and J. W. Hagen (Hillsdale, New Jersey: Erlbaum, 1977).

32. S. B. Messer, "Reflection-Impulsivity: A Review," *Psychological Bulletin* 83 (1976): 1026–52.

33. J. Piaget, *The Construction of Reality in the Child* (New York: Basic Books, 1954).

34. S. Hans, "Study of Self-Concept in Children" (Ph.D. diss., Harvard University, 1977).

35. Kagan, Kearsely, and Zelazo, *Infancy: Its Place* (See note 17).

36. J. Kagan and H. A. Moss, *Birth to Maturity* (New York: John Wiley, 1962).

37. J. Kagan, D. Lapidus, and M. Moore, "Infant Antecedents of Later Cognitive Functioning," *Child Development* 49 (1978): 1005–23.

38. M. Sigman and A. H. Parmelee, "Longitudinal Evaluation of the Pre-Term Infant," in *Infants Born at Risk,* ed. T. M. Field (New York: S. P. Medical and Scientific Books, 1979): 193–217, see esp. 215.

39. J. W. Macfarlane, "Perspectives in Personality Consistency and Change from the Guidance Study," *Vita Humana* 7 (1964): 115–26.

40. S. J. Suomi and H. F. Harlow, "Social Rehabilitation of Isolate-Reared Monkeys," *Developmental Psychology* 6 (1972): 487–96.

41. C. Rathbun, L. DiVirgilio, and S. Waldfogel, "The Restitutive Process in Children Following Radical Separation from Family and Culture," *American Journal of Orthopsychiatry* 28 (1958): 408–15, see esp. 413–14.

42. M. Winick, K. K. Meyer, and R. C. Harris, "Malnutrition and Environmental Enrichment by Early Adoption," *Science* 190 (1975): 1173–75.

43. W. Dennis, *Children of the Creche* (New York: Appleton-Century-Crofts, 1973).

44. J. Kagan, *Change and Continuity in Infancy* (New York: John Wiley, 1971).

45. Rutter, "Effects of Early Experience" (See note 24): 30.

46. J. McV. Hunt, "Psychological Development: Early Experience," in *Annual Review of Psychology,* vol. 30, ed. W. Porter and M. R. Rosenzweig (Palo Alto: California Annual Reviews, 1979).

47. M. Lewis and M. D. Starr, "Developmental Continuity," in *Handbook of Infant Development,* ed. J. D. Osofsky (New York: John Wiley, 1979): 653–70.

IMPACT ON ACADEMIC PEDIATRICS
OF PERINATAL MEDICINE

Michael A. Simmons

No subspecialty better characterizes the changes, succcsses, and uncertainties in academic pediatrics than the field of neonatal-perinatal medicine. Over the past fifteen years the subspecialty has been defined; a subspecialty board has been created; and clinical neonatal divisions have become among the most active in academic pediatrics departments. Neonatology as a specialty is presently encountering many difficulties, however, not only in the way it relates to the department of pediatrics, but within the specialty itself.

The theses I propose to develop are:

• Neonatology is a very nontraditional academic discipline; It has been defined by the collective, time-consuming clinical needs of an age-specific group of patients, not by a focused area of biology or pathology.

• The clinical needs of the patient population are so time-consuming that neonatology is progressively being identified only with clinical care. The results of that focus are not inconsequential: with the possible exception of the development of immunization and antibiotics, and the clear understanding of fluid and electrolyte disturbances in the diarrheal disorders, no disciplines has a more impressive record in reducing pediatric mortality and morbidity in the last twenty years than neonatology.

• Since the subspecialty is increasingly defined in purely

121

clinical terms, the neonatologist has become more of a generalist than a subspecialist, and generalists are still not easily incorporated into traditional academic structures.

• The service demands of the subspecialty have led to the proliferation of neonatology fellowship training programs in an effort to provide personnel to supervise the busy clinical services. Such service-oriented programs are, however, unlikely to produce graduates well adapted to or trained for a traditional academic career.

• There is currently no more exciting area of clinical pediatrics than the understanding and care of the prematurely born and other high-risk infants. There should be no higher priority for pediatricians than continuing to attack the problem of neonatal and infant mortality. If we are to be successful in reducing infant mortality and morbidity, we must continue to interest general pediatricians in the problems of the newborn and to train them in this area.

• The advances that will lead to the solution of neonatal and infant mortality problems during the 1980s are unlikely to be similar to those of the 1960s and 1970s. Solutions will come from a disciplined and focused attack on the biology, pathology, and pathophysiology of neonatal disorders and will require the involvement of specialties other than neonatology, at least as that subspecialty is currently constituted.

• Thus far there has been a disappointing involvement of academic disciplines—other than neonatology and pediatric cardiology—in the problems of the premature and other high-risk infants. Developing the interests of the other subspecialties in the biology and pathology of immaturity should be an important goal of the next decade.

PATIENT CARE

Patient care provisions in the newborn intensive care unit must be a major concern of successful departments of pediatrics. Table 1 outlines total pediatric patient days in four pediatric care facilities in various parts of the United States.

Hospital A is a general university teaching hospital.

Hospital B is a free-standing children's hospital in which a university teaching program is based; the department of

TABLE 1. PATIENT-CARE DAYS IN A VARIETY OF INPATIENT
PEDIATRIC FACILITIES IN THE UNITED STATES

	Total Patient Days	Nursery Days	Number of Faculty
Hospital A	65,000	19,000	4
Hospital B	70,000	12,000	6
With obstetrical beds	10,000	10,000	
Hospital C	49,000	13,000	6
With obstetrical beds	6,500	6,500	
Hospital D	30,000	11,000	6

NOTE: See text for a fuller explanation of the facilities of the four categories of hospitals.

pediatrics also supervises pediatric care in a maternity hospital that provides approximately 10,000 patient-care days a year.

Hospital C is a free-standing private children's hospital closely affiliated with the university teaching program; it also has an arrangement to provide coverage to a private obstetrical service in a community hospital.

Hospital D is a free-standing private children's hospital very loosely affiliated with a university teaching program.

Taking this quite varied sample of inpatient pediatric facilities as a whole, of the total pediatric inpatient days—excluding obstetrical hospital patient days—25 percent are accounted for by the nursery. If one includes patients who are the responsibility of the department of pediatrics, but whose care is delivered in an on-campus obstetrical hospital, 33 percent of total pediatric inpatient days are accounted for by the nursery. This is even more impressive when one consideres that a significant number of pediatric patient days are in fact surgical rather than medical admissions. It is therefore safe to assume that nearly 50 percent of inpatient pediatric medical days occur in the nursery. Thus neonatology services are essential to at least the financial survival of most pediatric hospitals.

The American Academy of Pediatrics (AAP), through its Committee on the Fetus and Newborn and Section on Perinatal Pediatrics, recently made a preliminary assessment of manpower needs in neonatology.[1] Based on its findings, as well as on estimates of the number of newborns requiring special care and the known number of neonatologists now certified, there is a nationwide shortfall of neonatologists, which is recognized in a variety of hospital settings throughout the country.

The foregoing assessment assumes that neonatologists provide services only in the intensive care setting. While models vary from one department to another, neonatologists are often responsible also for the organization and provision of services in full-term nurseries. There are alternatives to that model that make a great deal of sense. If we regard well-baby care as the beginning of a primary or continuing care process, rather than as a hospital-based function, this would lead to the incorporation of that responsibility into primary (ambulatory) care programs.

One response to meeting the demands for clinical service has been the escalation of neonatal fellowship training programs. Table 2, based on data from a survey made by the Ross Laboratories in Columbus, Ohio, shows that there are currently 175 neonatal training programs in the United States providing a total of 329 filled fellowship positions. There are potentially more fellowship positions available that are unfilled. Many of these fellowship programs are based in institutions that have no large house staff programs or functioning allied health programs, such as those for nurse clinicians or nurse practitioners. It is clear that the majority of the fellowship positions are primarily for the provision of service. Of the 329 fellows, for example, only twenty-eight have a primary laboratory commitment; an additional sixty-seven have had some laboratory experience associated with clinical research interests or projects.

In most traditional academic settings neonatal intensive

TABLE 2. NEONATAL FELLOWSHIP TRAINING PROGRAMS
IN THE UNITED STATES, 1980

Number of programs	175
Number of fellowship positions	329
Positions with laboratory commitments	28

SOURCE: Ross Laboratories, Columbus, Ohio.

care is primarily the responsibility of house staff. The Task Force on Pediatric Education has, however, recommended that the house staff experience in neonatal intensive care units be limited:

> Service demands for neonatal intensive care have frequently led to more lengthy residency experience in these units than is necessary to teach the core content. Almost half of pediatricians completing residencies since 1975 have felt that the training experience in newborn care was excessive. Forceful measures must be adopted to correct this imbalance in the educational program.[2]

Given the importance of newborn patient-care days to the financial integrity of pediatric hospitals and care facilities, it is important that academic pediatrics address the problem of how to meet service demands in such labor-intensive situations. The newborn intensive care unit is an example of an area where excellent clinical care is not provided because house staff or other practitioners are stationed there with loose or perfunctory once-a-day supervision by a faculty member. The challenge to academic pediatrics is to find ways of incorporating into the academic process neonatologists who have identified themselves as clinical care providers and allied health practitioners who increasingly will be needed to provide services to the newborn.

There has been some discussion during this meeting about financial compensation for neonatal faculty members, which is evidently higher than it is for other pediatric faculty. I suspect this may be true based on the weight of anecdotal evidence I have heard, but I have not seen firm data. I would argue that, if indeed neonatologists are compensated at a rate similar to that of faculty in internal medicine and to some in surgery, the solution is to increase the salaries of other pediatric faculty.

It is often assumed that neonatologists are able to collect substantial fees because the specialty is akin to a "surgical" specialty. I doubt this is the case. Leon Eisenberg has lamented the "procedure-related" nature of third-party reimbursement. I am familiar with such fee data on only one neonatal service. At Johns Hopkins less than 10 percent of our total professional fee income is "procedure-related," thus over 90 percent of our professional fee income reflects time spent with patients. Such fees would be as easily collected by any pediatrician as by a neonatal subspecialist.

TEACHING

Most of the teaching by neonatologists is directed toward postgraduate trainees (house staff). There is a growing recognition, however, that dependence on house staff to provide all required neonatal intensive care services can distort their educational experience.[3] But it would be a mistake to assume that experience in the neonatal intensive care unit is not pertinent to the training of a general pediatrician. According to the Task Force on Pediatric Education 25 percent of pediatricians trained since 1975 indicated that the amount of time spent in newborn care during their residencies was "excessive."[4] It is interesting to compare that response to the answer to the question about competency of the pediatrician to deal with various areas of her/his practice. These same respondents expressed more confidence in their ability to deal with newborn problems than with virtually any other area of pediatrics. To dismiss the importance of neonatal intensive care experience in the training of a general pediatrician would be to dismiss the importance of a pediatrician knowing how to care for a sick infant.

There has perhaps not been enough emphasis on the more generalized skills and knowledge that may be acquired during an experience in a newborn intensive care unit. In addition to learning specific neonatal disease processes and management techniques, the nature of the critical care environment requires a house officer to develop expertise in resuscitation; acid-base balance; fluid and electrolyte homeostasis; nutrition; pharmacology; clinical genetics; and the social-behavioral aspects of parenting. I suspect that nowhere in the pediatric curriculum are there more obvious and dramatic examples of proper and improper parenting than in a newborn intensive care unit. Learning about crisis management, parental attachment, and the care of a critically ill or dying child is routine in such an environment.

We should be concerned about the growing attitude that pediatricians should be trained to take care of well children rather than sick children. There has been too little emphasis on biosocial pediatrics, community health, and preventive health maintenance in traditional academic pediatrics departments. To assume the converse, however, that the care of sick children is not an important function of a pediatrician, as we enter the 1980s would be folly. Due largely to the successes of pediatrics in the past half-century, fewer older infants and children develop life-threatening diseases. It thus becomes extremely important to teach management approaches to life-threatening illness in those pediatric arenas where such problems are common; but there is really only one such area, and that is the newborn intensive care unit.

There is less of a role for medical students in newborn intensive care units. Without a solid background in general pediatrics the distractions therein can interfere with the educational process. If the focus of teaching could be on the easily observable aspects of growth, maturation, and development that occur in a newborn and in its family in the first few days of life, newborn medicine would be a potentially fertile area for the education of medical students.

Academic departments of pediatrics should make attempts to find ways to properly integrate students and their primary clerkships into a role that focuses on those aspects of the newborn course that relate to social-psychological adaptation, rather than concentrate solely on disease detection and management.

RESEARCH

It is ironic that the specialty of neonatology, which was created around a group of investigators, both clinical and laboratory, is now progressively practiced by individuals who have had little training in, exposure to, or interest in investigation. My personal estimate is that fewer than thirty of the 175 identified neonatology training programs have significant ongoing programs in laboratory research. Although there is no doubt that creative and scholarly clinical research can and does exist in the absence of a laboratory base, in my opinion most substantial clinical research in neonatalogy emanates from programs with a significant commitment to laboratory investigation.

The impact on fellowship training of a substantial laboratory or clinical research experience has two separate but related effects. First, in the absence of a research experience the fellow is deprived of training in reflective thought, problem definition, study design, and, one hopes, problem-solving skills. Second, neonatal faculty positions are potentially populated with persons who have had no research experience and no commitment to research as a career objective. Those same fellowship programs are thus staffed with faculty responsible for training new fellows; they are not interested in or capable of fostering a research component of a training program. We have already entered into this vicious circle of neonatology training.

The specialty has made such strides in the last fifteen years that lack of a generalized research base has thus far not had a severely deleterious impact. I suspect that the next few years will see us reach a plateau in the rate of progress that will occur in the application of current technology to clinical problems. We are now at a phase where new and basic information is needed.

If an ultimate aim is to reduce the number of premature infants, we need a better understanding of the mechanisms of parturition. Our present approach to premature rupture of membranes and premature labor is crude and relatively ineffective. We should not even be sanguine that the ability to interrupt labor is desirable. There are at present a variety of tocolytic agents that have been proven effective; yet there is no evidence that tocolysis leads to any positive effect on pregnancy outcome.

In order to understand the biology of immaturity, more attention needs to be devoted to all aspects of developmental biology—developmental chemistry, developmental physiology, and developmental pharmacology. We have enough information to lead to a recognition that developing organisms, organs, tissues, and cells may be different than their mature counterparts.

We need more insightful and detailed descriptions of normal and abnormal fetal and neonatal growth characteristics. Disturbances in growth (size and maturity) account for most infant mortality and morbidity rates. We have only the most rudimentary understanding of implantation, placentation, and early embryology. Although there are many detailed descriptive studies of fetal physiology in the last quarter of pregnancy, features of early fetal physiology are entirely unknown. We know little concerning the mechanisms that control fetal growth. In particular, detailed investigative attention should be given to those organs such as the lungs and the brain whose dysfunction accounts for the high rates of acute mortality and long-term morbidity.

We know little of the physiology of the immature neonate. Although the last fifteen years have seen the emergence of some information concerning respiratory and circulatory physiology of premature infants, we know little of the renal physiology, gastrointestinal physiology, and neurophysiology of immature neonates.

Norman Kretchmer stated earlier in this conference that support for nutritional research is a high priority of the National Institute of Child Health and Human Development. There is no area that has more direct relevance to or is of such basic biological importance to the care of premature infants than nutrition. The present approach to the nutrition of the low-birth-weight infant is embarassingly primitive.

There remains in neonatal medicine much opportunity for creative clinical research. Neonatal management issues, particularly as they relate to specific long-term outcome, require systematic testing. Concern about abnormal parenting, which appears to occur commonly in families with premature infants, likewise needs critical dissection.

I am skeptical about whether the solution to these problems will come from the specialty of neonatology alone. If scholarship and creativity require time for thought and reflection, an educational and training background on which to build, discipline, and intramural and extramural financial support, then neonatology as a specialty is likely to be found lacking in its ability to solve most of the problems outlined. But, in contrast to the other specialties, it has at least demonstrated a definitive interest in these areas. The challenge is to find a way to involve other more traditional academic disciplines in the biological problems of immaturity and the clinical problems of sick newborns.

Perhaps this is not a forum for recommendations, but I

would suggest we consider neonatal fellowship training as having two distinct parts. First would be the acquisition of the clinical knowledge and technical skills required for care of critically ill infants; the time-consuming nature and underlying importance of this knowledge and these skills should not be underestimated. The second component would be a scholarly or creative one. When a basic laboratory environment or a basic interest in clinical research does not exist within a neonatal division, one attractive possibility would be to provide this experience in other active laboratories within the academic department. This would serve not only to give neonatal fellows experience in a rigorous research environment, but begin to interest other academic disciplines in the problems of immature and other high-risk infants. This is obviously not a new model, but one that has been tried to some extent in several pediatrics departments. A major constraint has been the lack of time because of service demands that are built into so many neonatal fellowship training programs.

SUMMARY

• Academic pediatrics must encourage the development of new ways to provide service to high-risk infants and to integrate and accept faculty members, whether they are M.D.'s, nurses, or allied health practitioners, whose primary function is the clinical care of high-risk infants.

• The newborn intensive care unit provides one of the few arenas in pediatrics where principles of critical care can be taught efficiently. Care of the critically ill child is an important aspect of pediatric training.

• Over the next decade the existing clinical dilemmas in neonatal pediatrics are unlikely to yield, as they have in the past, to the simple application of current technology.

• A rapidly expanding investigation base focused on a biological understanding of immaturity is essential, but it is unlikely to come solely from the discipline of neonatology.

• Other academic disciplines within departments of pediatrics must be encouraged to become interested in the biology of immaturity and in the problems of high-risk new-borns.

• Academic departments must begin to take some respon-sibility for the curriculum of neonatal fellowship training pro-grams. It should be the department's responsibility to balance the service and educational components of neonatal fellowship training so that the young neonatologists who will populate our academic departments in the near future have the educational background and the training experience that will make re-search an exciting and indispensable part of their career objec-tives. A research experience during fellowship training will, at the minimum, make a clinician more scholarly in his approach to patient care.

Notes

1. Committee on Fetus and Newborn and Section on Perinatal Pediatrics, Amer-ican Academy of Pediatrics, "Estimates of Need and Recommendations for Personnel in Neonatal Pediatrics," *Pediatrics* 65 (1980): 850–53.

2. *The Future of Pediatric Education, Report of the Task Force on Pediatric Education* (Evanston, Illinois: Task Force on Pediatric Education, nd [1978?]).

3. Ibid.

4. Ibid.

IMPACT ON ACADEMIC PEDIATRICS
OF CONCEPTS IN INFANT NUTRITION

Ilene Fennoy

Nutrition is a body of science concerned with the relationship of foodstuffs to the growth, development, and maintenance of the organism. As such it includes biochemical and physiological concepts that relate to every field of medicine.[1]

The entire field of growth and development, with its emphasis on the well-being of the child, is of primary concern to pediatrics; thus pediatrics and nutrition have been intimately linked through the years. In this paper I will focus on several aspects of infant nutrition that are of particular relevance to growth and development, and on some of the concepts learned in the course of such research that may guide our future progress.

Historically there has been much concern over the appropriate feeding of infants.[2-4] A rational basis for the choice of infant food, however, awaited the linking of the nutritional, chemical, and physiological sciences. This link began with Antoine L. Lavoisier's discovery of oxygen in 1777 and progressed through François Magendie's proof in the early nineteenth century that all animals must have organic forms of nitrogen in their food.[5] By the nineteenth century the groundwork had therefore been laid for a practical and experimental approach to nutrition, and the concept of caloric requirements as a basis of nutrition could be pursued.

With the beginning of the twentieth century came the

recognition of essential elements in the diet, particularly the vitamins.[6] The sources of deficiency diseases such as scurvy, rickets, and pellagra were resolved early in this century.[7]

The interest in vitamin deficiency syndromes not only led to the discovery of their cause and the dietary source of the curative factors, but to the synthetic production of these substances. This achievement of vitamin synthesis is a particularly important factor in the prevention of vitamin deficiency, for it provides the possibility of widespread supplementation of staple foods.[8] Thus today we have infant formulas with multivitamin supplements and breads and cereals with vitamin B supplements.[9] As a result we seldom see vitamin deficiency syndromes in routine clinical pediatric practice in the United States.

The emphasis on vitamins became so great that in 1921 R. McCarrison in his book, *Studies in Deficiency Disease*, stated that although

> vitamins have their place in nutrition, it is that of one link in a chain of essential substances requisite for the harmonious regulation of the chemical process of healthy cellular action.[10]

Nevertheless, the interest in deficiency diseases, particularly as they related to vitamins, continued. In the early 1930s, when Cicely D. Williams described protein malnutrition, or kwashiorkor—"the disease of the deposed infant"[11-13]—her theory was hotly contested by other researchers, who claimed the condition was a form of pellagra. It was several years before the concept of protein deficiency as the cause of kwashiorkor was accepted.[14,15] Subsequent investigations of the biochemical basis of protein malnutrition revealed that the quality, as well as the quantity, of a substance is important in nutrition.

Examples of this concept are seen when the value of corn protein versus milk protein is studied relative to the needs of the infant and the adult. The infant requires nine amino acids instead of the usual eight because of its need for histidine. In addition, the total required amounts of these amino acids in milligrams per gram of protein is greater for the infant than for the adult.[16,17] Thus a protein with the eight essential amino acids, but without histidine, is qualitively poor for the infant, although adequate for the adult. Moreover the protein is no better than its most limiting amino acid, that is, even with all nine essential amino acids a protein lacking a sufficient quantity of one amino acid to meet the individual's need will be inadequate.[18]

Recognition of such deficiencies within a protein has led to supplementation of cereal protein with specific amino acids to improve its quality, or to the combination of several proteins to achieve a balance of amino acids.[19-21] This technique has proved valuable in generating better quality foods without radical alteration of local dietary patterns, thereby alleviating some of the malnutrition seen in growing children.[22,23]

Trace mineral research is another area of nutrition study that has blossomed in recent years.[24] Clinical interest was aroused by the increasing use of synthetic diets, especially total parenteral nutrition (TPN),[25] in which deficiency states rapidly become obvious. Further evaluation led to the recognition of trace minerals as important elements in enzyme systems, as cofactors for metal-iron activated enzymes, and as essential constituents of other important molecules.[26]

This research led to the treatment of new syndromes of particular relevance to pediatricians, with our increased capability of maintaining the premature and dysmature infant. Not only are we now aware of mineral deficiency syndromes, but of the interaction of one nutrient with another. A number of minerals—copper and zinc, for example—have been studied particularly thoroughly and serve to illustrate some of the concepts emerging from this line of research.

Copper deficiency has been described in the premature infant or in the baby over age six months fed exclusively on a diet of cow's milk—a poor source of copper.[27] In addition, the deficiency is seen in the genetic syndrome of decreased copper absorption known as Menkes' steely hair disease, as well as in diseases associated with chronic diarrhea. Manifestations initially include anemia and osteoporosis, followed by failure to thrive, skin lesions, anorexia, and diarrhea; treatment consists in the administration of copper sulfate. For premature infants copper-supplemented formulas are recommended as a means of prevention; for the full-term infant, progress to a mixed diet by age six months usually avoids the problem.

Copper is important as a constituent of several enzymes such as cytochrome oxidase and ceruloplasmin.[28] The latter acts as a ferroxidase, thereby facilitating iron absorption and release from the reticuloendothelial system. Oxidation of iron is necessary for binding to transferrin and transport to bone marrow. Thus copper is important for iron utilization, with a deficiency manifesting itself as an anemia similar to that of iron deficiency. Here the concept of nutrient interaction is exemplified.

Zinc is another mineral about which we have gained much clinically useful data: it is associated with a genetic syndrome of a defect in zinc absorption—acrodermatitis enterohepatica—as well as inadequate dietary intake.[29] Clinical manifestations include growth retardation, alteration in the sense of taste, alopecia, and delayed sexual maturation. Meat protein is the best source of zinc and is associated with the most complete absorption; vegetables and dairy products are generally low in zinc. Reports of diets supplemented with zinc, but not copper, suggest that zinc interferes with copper absorption and leads to an elevated serum cholesterol.[30] Whether this reflects a simple imbalance of nutrients or an actual adverse effect of one nutrient on another remains controversial.[31] Nevertheless the zinc-copper interaction is an example of the concept that one nutrient interacts with another and affects absorption and utilization.[32]

The concept of nutrient interaction has been clearly identified in the premature infant in terms of vitamin E, polyunsaturated fatty acids (PUFA), and iron. With the use of infant formulas high in PUFA, a vitamin E-dependent hemolytic anemia has been shown to develop.[33,34] Prevention and treatment may be achieved by supplementing these PUFA-rich infant formulas with vitamin E. In the presence of iron-supplemented formula, however, the response to vitamin E supplementation is poor; the iron depresses the absorption of vitamin E.[35] Thus if the premature infant ingests a PUFA-rich formula it is not only at risk for iron deficiency anemia, but for hemolytic anemia secondary to vitamin E deficiency. Formula supplements must be geared to meet these competing demands.

In recent years it has become clear that nutritional status

has implications for other aspects of health besides growth and development. For example, current studies show that immunological status is dependent on nutritional well-being.[36] Even in the otherwise healthy, breast-fed, versus formula-fed, infant one may find a lower incidence of allergy and a less frequent illness history because of the immune factors present in breast milk.[37]

At present our interest is no longer focused on the deficiency states, except in high-risk cases such as premature infants or those with chronic diarrhea. We are becoming increasingly concerned about excess intakes of nutrients, particularly with respect to calories, fat, and cholesterol. This concept of such excesses being associated with disease states, although recognized by nutritionists for years, is becoming widely accepted.[38]

In order to minimize the likelihood of coronary artery disease adults are being urged by the American Heart Association (AHA) to adopt a "prudent diet," that is, one with less than 300 mg. of cholesterol per day; less than 35 percent of total calories from fat and less than 10 percent from saturated fats; and to maintain their ideal body weight.[39]

These recommendations are causing much controversy among pediatricians. Part of the controversy concerns the lack of evaluation of the AHA-recommended diets with respect to other parameters of well-being related to growth and development. Such diets have been fairly extensively evaluated in the population at risk for coronary heart disease, and little evidence of adversity has been demonstrated. This group does not, however, represent the large population of children on marginal diets.[40] What are the implications for these children of a reduction in fat intake, particularly saturated fat, which comes primarily from meat proteins, which are one of the better sources of trace minerals. With recommendations for meat restriction, will the marginal diets of these children be adequate for optimal growth and development?

Such questions relating to the interaction of nutrients, the balance of nutrients, and requirements specific for age relate to the basic principles of nutrition mentioned earlier. These include the facts that: 1) deficiency diseases exist; 2) requirements are specific for age and circumstance; 3) the quality of a nutrient, as well as its quantity, is of importance; and 4) nutrient interactions occur that may interface with ultimate utilization. If we are to optimize our diet these principles must not be forgotten in our goal to remedy nutrient excess.

In summary, then, it is evident from the examples I have cited that nutrition plays a key role in improving the health and well-being of our children. Yet if this role is to continue, and if we are to answer the questions of the future, we must ensure a place for nutrition both in pediatric research and in the education of the pediatric house officer.

The questions in nutrition research today are as significant for health as at any time in the past. The information at our disposal and that being generated from current research is detailed and complex. It will take a well-organized, systematic program of instruction to impart this information to pediatricians in training if they are to use it optimally in behalf of their patients and generate the answers of the future.

NOTES

1. C. R. Gallagher and V. M. Vivian, "Nutrition Concepts Essential in the Education of the Medical Student," *American Journal of Clinical Nutrition* 32 (June 1979): 1330–33.

2. I. G. Wickes, "A History of Infant Feeding. Part III: Eighteenth and Nineteenth Century Writers," *Archives of the Diseases of Childhood* 28 (1953): 332–40.

3. ———, "A History of Infant Feeding. Part IV: Nineteenth Century Continued," ibid.: 416–422.

4, ———, "A History of Infant Feeding. Part V: Nineteenth Century Concluded and Twentieth Century," ibid.: 495–502.

5 H. H. Williams, "The Founding of the American Institute of Nutrition, Including Commentaries on the Founders," *Federation Proceedings* 36, no. 6 (May 1977): 1915–18.

6. E. N. Todhunter, "Some Classics of Nutrition and Dietetics," *Journal of the American Dietetic Association* 44 (February 1964): 100–08.

7. E. V. McCollum, "The End of an Era: New Horizons," in *A History of Nutrition* (Boston: Houghton Mifflin Co., 1957): 420–23.

8. W. H. Sebrell, Jr., "Clinical Nutrition in the United States. IV." *American Journal of Public Health* 58, no. 11 (November 1968): 2035–42.

9. A. E. Bender, "Manufactured Foods," in *Textbook of Pediatric Nutrition*, ed. D. S. McClaren and D. Burman (New York: Churchill Livingston, 1976): 375–86.

10. R. McCarrison, *Studies in Deficiency Disease* (London: Oxford Medical Publications, 1921).

11. C. D. Williams, "Deficiency Diseases in Infants," in *Annual Medical Report of the Gold Coast for 1931 and 1932*. (1932): 93; repr. in *Nutrition Review* 31, no. 11 (November 1973): 341–43.

12. ———, "A Nutritional Disease of Childhood Associated with a Maize Diet," *Archives of Diseases in Childhood* 8 (1933): 423, repr. in ibid.: 344–49.

13. ———, "Kwashiorkor: A Nutritional Disease of Children Associated with a Maize Diet," *Lancet* 2 (16 November 1935): 1151; repr. in ibid.: 350–51.

14. ———, "The Study of Kwashiorkor," *Courrier* (Centre International de l'Enfance, Paris) XIII, no. 6 (1963): repr. in ibid.: 334–40.

15. H. C. Trowell, J. N. P. Davies, and R. F. A. Dean, "The History of Kwashiorkor," in *Kwashiorkor*, pt. 2 (London: Edward Arnold, Ltd. 1954): 12–47.

16. G. Arroyave, "Amino Acid Requirements and Age," in *Protein-Calorie Malnutrition*, ed. R. E. Olson (New York: Academic Press, 1975): 1–22.

17. Food and Nutrition Board, *Evaluation of Protein Quality*, publ. no. 1100 (Washington: National Academy of Sciences/National Research Council, 1963).

18. Arroyave, "Amino Acid Requirements" (See note 16).

19. Ibid.

20. Food and Nutrition Board, *Protein Quality* (See note 17).

21. Bender, "Manufactured Foods" (See note 9).

22. Arroyave, "Amino Acid Requirements" (See note 16).

23. Bender, "Manufactured Foods" (See note 9).

24. E. J. Underwood, "The History and Philosophy of Trace Element Research," in *Newer Trace Elements in Nutrition*, ed. W. Mertz and W. E. Cornatzer (New York: Marcel Dekker, Inc., 1971): 1–18.

25. K. M. Hambidge, "Trace Elements in Pediatric Nutrition," *Advances in Pediatrics* 24 (1977): 191–231.

26. Ibid.

27. Ibid.

28. Ibid.

29. Ibid.

30. Ibid.

31. Ibid.

32. D. M. Hegsted, "Interactions in Nutrition," in *Newer Trace Elements in Nutrition*, ed. W. Mertz and W. E. Cornatzer (New York: Marcel Dekker, Inc., 1971): 19–32.

33. D. K. Melhorn and S. Gross, "Vitamin E-Dependent Anemia in the Premature Infant. I. Effects of Large Doses of Medicinal Iron," *Journal of Pediatrics* 79, no. 4 (October 1971): 569–80.

34. ———, "Vitamin E-Dependent Anemia in the Premature Infant. II. Relationships Between Gestational Age and Absorption of Vitamin E," in ibid.: 581–88.

35. Ibid.

36. R. K. Chandra, "Interactions of Nutrition, Infection and Immune Response," *Acta Paediatrica Scandinavica* 68 (1979): 137–44.

37. Committee on Nutrition, American Academy of Pediatrics, "Breast-Feeding," *Pediatrics* 62, no. 4 (October 1978): 591–601.

38. "Report of the Inter-Society Commission for Heart Disease Resources," *Circulation* 42 (December 1970): A55–95.

39. Ibid.

40. "Highlights from the Ten-State Nutrition Survey," *Nutrition Today* (July/August 1972): 4–11.

IMPACT ON ACADEMIC PEDIATRICS OF HUMAN GENETICS: PAST, PRESENT, PROSPECTS, AND PROBLEMS

John W. Littlefield

A few years ago I was visiting the dean of a large medical school that had a substantial cancer research program, and he declared: "First we are going to conquer cancer and then we will take on genetics!" Clearly the battle with genetics was going to be on a large and magnificent scale, and clearly the outcome was inevitable—the elimination of genetics as a "problem"! Although I have been more of an observer of than a participant in genetics in recent years, the perspective of that dean reaffirmed my belief that genetics will refuse to be eliminated! You may legitimately remind me of the apt quotation, "If your only tool is a hammer, you begin to think that every problem is a nail," but I still insist that genetics is here to stay because it underlies all of medicine!

THE PAST

In the 1950s medical geneticists were often believed to be preoccupied with exotic problems: "If you hear hoofbeats in the distance, call it a zebra before you call it a horse!" The field was frequently referred to as "genetic counseling."

Medical genetics as we know it today emerged about twenty years ago with the confluence of several gentle streams:

139

biochemical genetics, immunogenetics, population genetics, cytogenetics, and clinical genetics.

Biochemical genetics originated in the late 1940s with the electrophoretic studies of Linus Pauling and others on sickle cell hemoglobin, and the development by Dent and others of chromatographic techniques to separate the amino acids found in the urine of certain mentally retarded individuals, and then to separate the peptides contained in hemoglobins and other blood proteins.

Immunogenetics emerged shortly after the turn of the century with studies of blood groups; it achieved its greatest practical result a few years ago with the prevention of Rh disease.

Population genetics first appeared in England many years ago. Today it is represented in practice by genetic screening programs aimed initially at affected individuals, and then at those whose genes pose a risk for their offspring.

Clinical genetics began as a tranquil, anecdotal, largely descriptive subspecialty with little therapeutic importance. What energized clinical genetics about twenty years ago was the sudden emergence of cytogenetics, which provided a simple and rapid method to analyze the complement of chromosomes of a given individual. The chromosomal bases of Down's syndrome, Klinefelter's syndrome, and Turner's syndrome were quickly established, and as a result human genetics got its own tissue and its legitimacy as a medical subspecialty.

If cytogenetics introduced the modern era of medical genetics, about ten years ago geneticists acquired a remarkable new tool—prenatal genetic diagnosis. This technique opened a "window" on the fetus halfway through gestation, allowing identification of its sex and chromosome complement, and a glimpse of its enzymes, its blood, and even some of its anatomy. The ability to predict features of an unborn child reassures many parents worried about the possibility of a genetic disorder. I believe parents want to know as much about their offspring before birth as can safely be elicited, and indeed they have the right to have this information.

But people to some extent still confuse the remarkable medical advances of prenatal genetic diagnosis with the much less clear-cut issue of abortion for social reasons. More broadly, prenatal diagnosis and other advances in genetics have forced society to begin to deal with the ramifications of modern biomedical technology. For eventually it is all of society, not just physicians and scientists, that must put into proper perspective the social, legal, and ethical aspects of modern medicine.

THE PRESENT

Several studies have shown that among children admitted to a referral pediatric hospital, 10 to 20 percent are there for the treatment of disorders with a clear genetic basis, and another 10 to 20 percent for developmental malformations, which, in our present state of ignorance, may often have a genetic basis. Add to this group of children with obvious or probable genetic disorders the potent effect of heredity on the susceptibility to other diseases, on behavioral problems, and on health in general, and it is clear that genetics is of central importance to pediatrics. Furthermore it is now widely appreciated that genetics extends across adult medicine, underlying the susceptibility to many common disorders. We have come to realize that each person is genetically unique, a concept first suggested by Sir Archibald Garrod; an episode of disease is the result of the interaction between a unique individual and a specific environment.

Medical genetics has assumed many responsibilities in recent years. Genetics and endocrinology share patients with metabolic diseases, although genetics tends to be more concerned with the inborn metabolic errors of the newborn. A striking development in recent years has been the demonstration of extensive genetic heterogeneity in practically all inborn errors of metabolism examined in detail. Examples are the glycogen storage and lipid storage diseases, the inherited hemolytic anemias, and such seemingly simple conditions as maple syrup urine disease and phenylketonuria.

Geneticists are also responsible for the evaluation of children with malformations involving more than one organ, especially the complex congenital malformation syndromes, of which several hundred are now recognized. A few professionals with much experience and unusual memories of the constellations of signs in these syndromes seem to be confident about the diagnosis of each one; others of us are bewildered by the possibilities. Only a few physical abnormalities are quantifiable as yet, so one cannot be sure that each feature is definitely present.

We urgently need a way out of this situation! Better methods must be developed to standardize and compare many different measurements of the face, the head, and the extremities, for example, as well as a computer program to rank the likely diagnostic possibilities. This will give us more confidence in the classification of the congenital malformation syndromes, but it will not of course clarify their etiologies. Here progress in the identification of chromosomal, epidemiological, teratogenic, and pharmacogenetic factors may be helpful.

One of the surprises of our era has been the frequency with which chromosomal aberrations occur. These usually lead to miscarriage, but about one in 200 pregnancies results in a viable infant with a serious chromosomal abnormality. Over the past decade the development of several chromosomal banding techniques has given much added precision to chromosomal diagnosis, permitting specific identification of each chromosome and localization to regions thereof. A recent improvement concentrates on chromosomes in prophase, when they are especially stretched. Also, mostly through the techniques of somatic cell genetics, over 350 genes have been assigned to specific individual chromosomes—a third of them to the X chromosome, which attracts attention because of the unusual pattern of inheritance it produces. It is truly remarkable that in the past few years an extensive human chromosome map has been constructed that now equals the mouse chromosome map in complexity!

Finally, geneticists are primarily responsible for the expanding programs of genetic screening; for genetic counseling concerning the likelihood of disease in offspring; and, in concert with obstetricians, for prenatal genetic diagnosis. Some of the first direct applications of modern molecular genetics to clinical medicine are appearing in the prenatal diagnosis of sickle-cell anemia and thalassemia through identification of common variations in the structure of DNA segments near the hemoglobin gene.

Indeed medical geneticists seem to be waiting in eager anticipation for the results of the flood of current research concerning the structure of genes in eukaryotic cells. This work is based on the discovery ten years ago of enzymes called "site-specific restriction endonucleases," which cleave DNA into specific pieces. With the help of other enzymes these pieces can be introduced into viruses or other transmissable genetic elements, which can then be used to infect bacteria, or even animal cells. In this way the single piece of DNA can be multiplied a billion times overnight, allowing the study of individual genes of the mammalian chromosome that were previously unapproachable because they are so rare. The human genome contains 1 million to 10 million such genes and is 1,000 times more complex than that of *E. coli,* which in turn is 1,000 times more complex than that of the SV40 virus. These new recombinant DNA techniques have finally broken the logjam in our understanding of the molecular structure and function of the chromosome, thus producing a true revolution in biology in recent years.

Before long we should see the first fruits of this new technology; human insulin, growth hormone, and interferon produced through these techniques should soon be available. More important, we can anticipate steady progress in our understanding of how gene expression is controlled and how the mysterious process of development is programmed. Completely unexpected properties of genes have already been discovered, including the presence of seemingly inactive segments that must be removed prior to "read out." Certain genes on separate chromosomes must be brought together physically in order to function. Other genes are known to be duplicated, in some cases many times.

We are beginning to recognize that genes may exist "on the loose" in animal cells, as in bacteria. Techniques have been developed to transfer chromosomes and even single genes between animal cells. The most precise of these techniques involves the injection of a gene directly into the nucleus of a cell through a microneedle! Given this development, who would deny that it will become possible to replace abnormal genes in a human being? Indeed it was reported very recently that a new gene had been introduced into mouse cells in culture, and that these cells were subsequently made to repopulate a mouse!

PROSPECTS

At the present rapid pace certain achievements seem likely to occur in medical genetics in the next decade or two.

The locations of the genes for most of the proteins known to be present in a human cell will probably be assigned to regions of specific chromosomes, which will be delineated more and more specifically by new banding techniques. Many regulatory proteins, and those appearing only during development, will begin to be mapped in the same way. The detailed molecular structure, including coding and noncoding regions and the flanking regions on both sides, will be characterized for many normal and mutant genes. As a result the mechanisms of control and function of genes will be understood in detail, including the activation of certain genes only during development.

Enzyme therapy, that is, the replacement of missing enzymes, may become commonplace—perhaps the mainstay of treatment for storage diseases. These techniques may in some way be extended to some of the degenerative diseases of the central nervous system. Further down the road will be the insertion of "new" genes into individuals—and that time may not be so far off as some of us once thought. It was only a few years ago that Maurice Fox and I wrote, in reference to genetic engineering, "We must not do to ourselves what we have done to our environment!" The potentially harmful side effects of human genetic engineering are still of much concern, but the likelihood that it will occur now seems certain. The first attempts will probably involve genetic manipulation of a person's own cells in culture, followed by reinjection, unless it becomes possible to overcome present histocompatibility barriers.

Within a decade or two much progress should be made concerning our knowledge of the mechanisms of normal development and the ways in which it can go wrong. Here the intellectual gulf between the laboratory and the clinic is currently very broad and deep. Doubtless we will come to recognize many teratogens, carcinogens, and mutagens in our environment of which we are now unaware.

Genetic screening programs will continue to increase, particularly when prenatal diagnosis is available for the trait under study. The scope of prenatal diagnosis should expand with the identification of more genes that are inactive in amniotic fluid cells through the use of polymorphisms in neighboring DNA or through the activation of these genes. We should be able to identify specifically those individuals who are particularly at risk for certain malignancies, for arteriosclerotic heart disease, for hypertension, or for pharmacogenetic problems, as well as for deficiencies in host-defense mechanisms that cause especial susceptibility to infections.

Finally, we can hope for progress in our understanding of the multigenic inheritance of common disorders, with identification of the genes culminating in such inheritance and the mechanisms by which they act. The uncommon "single-gene" traits leading to malformations, tumors, diabetes, and arteriosclerotic heart diseases, for example, should be studied first, because they hold much promise for our understanding of the common multigenic forms of these disorders, which are inherited in complex fashion involving the interaction of several genes and the environment.

THE PROBLEMS

With such a vivid and exciting potential future in mind I need to express concern about several likely obstacles. These relate to education, to research support, and to a wiser definition of roles in research.

First, I encounter, as others surely do, considerable ambivalence among people outside genetics about where the field is headed. Genetics has a more central, personal connotation than other subspecialties, except perhaps those dealing with the brain; this makes its advances more intriguing, but at the same time more alarming. We need a better process of continuing education for the public and for most scientists if we are to avoid prolonged future debates such as that concerning recombinant DNA. Continuing genetic education should also encourage the public and the professionals to make greater efforts to deal with the many ethical and legal issues that are now or will soon arise from the applications of genetic research.

Second, as in all areas of medical research we must resolve the problem of financial support to avoid the difficulties, unevenness, and disillusionments of the past decade. In addition to concern over the unpredictability of the administration and the Congress, there are questions about the efficiency and the success of current national mechanisms for the support of biomedical research. Perhaps we should look at the English system, under which, at least to an outsider, research grants seem to be awarded more simply, more quickly, and more consistently. Also, perhaps we should press for larger, longer, and less restricted support from American industry.

Finally, I am concerned about who will be doing genetic research in the future. From watching the development of recombinant DNA technology during recent years, both through the Recombinant DNA Advisory Committee and in our own laboratory, it is clear that this sort of work cannot be carried on in a part-time fashion. I expect that only rare and carefully selected people will become truly competent both in the practice of medicine and in genetic research in the years ahead, except when the problems studied are primarily clinical in nature. In this situation there is an opportunity for a more extensive and healthy partnership than has existed in the past between individuals with Ph.D. degrees and those with M.D. degrees. And, of course, there have always been personality traits more appropriate for one profession than the other!

Thus I suspect that the concept of the "physician-scientist," so strongly promoted in the 1950s and 1960s, is becoming outmoded for much of genetic research and perhaps for other areas. It is inevitable and desirable that genetic research should become so complex as to require full-time attention, and here again this will probably be true for other subspecialties. The problem will be to create a harmonious partnership between the physician, who will recognize a clinical problem and encourage the study of it in the laboratory, and the Ph.D.-scientist, who will be better equipped to carry out the study. For research to be productive, each individual must recognize with satisfaction his/her own contribution to a team effort; none should feel inferior. Human genetics may have an unusual opportunity in this regard, since in many schools it is already so organized as to bridge the gap between the basic sciences and the clinical departments.

IMPACT ON ACADEMIC PEDIATRICS
OF DEVELOPMENTAL NEUROBIOLOGY

Dominick P. Purpura

Developmental neurobiology is concerned with defining the principles underlying the developmental organization of nervous systems.[1] It seeks to elucidate the fundamental mechanisms of neurogenesis; how neurons migrate from their birthplace to their correct locations in the brain; what strategies ensure the establishment of appropriate synaptic relations; and, perhaps most important from the standpoint of human development, how the immature brain acquires the ability to learn and to attain wisdom.

Developmental neurobiology is not a discipline in the traditional sense. Rather it is a *way of thinking* about the ultimate biological enigma—how the brain works. The neurobiologist is by nature a multidisciplinarian. The *problem* is foremost and it dictates the extent to which anatomical, psychological, biochemical, and other operational approaches are combined to achieve a particular solution. In a certain sense neurobiology may be considered a biological growth industry, as is evidenced by the almost logarithmic growth of the neuroscience community over the past two decades and the increasing number of periodicals, new academic departments, and national and international societies devoted to neuroscience research.

What accounts for this extraordinary interest in and preoccupation with brain mechanisms? The answer may be sought in the expectation that the more one studies the structure and function of excitable membranes, the bioenergetics of neurons, the mechanisms of synaptic actions, the biochemical pharmacology of different neuronal circuits, and the manner in which indentifiable neuronal subsystems participate in simple behaviors, the more attractive becomes the likelihood of understanding even the most complex of human behaviors, including the mechanisms of "mind." Such optimism derives in part from recent discoveries and the development of powerful new techniques for probing the molecular as well as the molar organization of the brain. There are good reasons to believe that much of this new knowledge will have a profound impact on academic pediatrics, particularly those aspects concerned with disorders of neurobehavioral development.

Perhaps one of the more startling revelations to emanate from recent attempts to apply developmental neuroscience approaches to studies of the immature human brain is that developmental processes have advanced considerably by the middle of the last trimester of gestation. Observations reported from different laboratories have established that morphologically identifiable synapses are present in the primitive cerebral cortex of the human embryo by eight weeks![2] By six months the human fetal cerebrum probably contains *all* the neurons it will ever have, whereas the cerebellum continues to add neurons, largely small granule cells, throughout the first two postnatal years.[3,4]

Studies in laboratory animals have provided evidence that neurogenetic cycles are highly programmed and result in temporospatial patterns of neurons whose phenotypic features are related in part to their "birthdate," final address in the brain, and the influence of environmental, particularly local, neuronal relations. The fact that temporally overlapping developmental events may be modified at different stages by a variety of perturbations is now well established in studies of laboratory animals.

The translation of these findings into studies of developmental abnormalities of immature human brain is well underway. Because of the relevance of these observations to problems of perinatology it is useful to summarize them briefly.

The cerebral cortex of the twenty-four-week-old human

fetus contains virtually its full complement of neurons, but is deficient in glial cells whose numbers will increase to staggering proportions later, well into the postnatal period.[5] Although cortical neurons have attained their proper "address" by midgestation, they lack the complex dendritic systems and axonal collaterals that characterize mature neurons. The last trimester is particularly important in this regard, for it is within the relatively narrow time frame of between twenty-four and thirty-two weeks that neurons acquire their initial dendritic systems and establish major branching patterns.

The importance of this period, during which neurons synthesize and incorporate a relatively enormous mass of membrane into expanding processes to provide postsynaptic receptor surfaces, cannot be overemphasized. It is now known that metabolic, genetic, traumatic, and infectious processes that affect the fetus or preterm infant in this period of rapid dendritic growth and differentiation will produce grave abnormalities in dendritic architecture.[6] These abnormalities not only affect dendritic segment lengths and branching patterns, but have an impact on the number, morphology, and distribution of fine dendritic processes, termed *dendritic spines,* which are postsynaptic targets for the vast majority of synapses made on pyramidal neurons and other neurons with prominent spines.

The academic pediatrician should be aware of neurobiological data on synaptogenesis in the immature brain because much of what students, young house officers, and clinical research fellows learn about pediatric medicine, such as inborn errors of metabolism, renal dysfunction, or cardiopulmonary diseases, has a direct or indirect effect on the most delicate and vulnerable of growth processes—the formation of appropriate synaptic relations between neurons.

One of the truly awesome biological statistics is that during human brain maturation 200 billion neurons will be generated, develop, and make appropriate synaptic connections such that each neuron will receive from 10,000 to 200,000 synaptic connections and will make the same number or more synapses with other neurons, including some with itself! Were this all the developmental neurobiologist had to contend with it would be difficult, but not impossible, to catalogue most synaptic relations utilizing established neurophysiological and light and electron microscopic studies of "classical" synaptic pathways.

What now appears to be a major confounding factor in developmental synaptology is that much of the chemical signaling between neurons may involve agents that are not released at "classical" synapses such as the neuromuscular junction. Further it is clear that chemical modulation of neuronal function may have widespread effects on the excitability of large populations of neurons—effects that persist for minutes, hours, days, and perhaps longer! Contrast this with the "classical," rapid and brief synaptic action of acetylcholine at the skeletal neuromuscular junction; effects that have provided and continue to provide the basic principles of synaptic operations.

Developmental neurobiology must now incorporate a huge volume of new data indicating that neurons may utilize a wide variety of chemical agents, including amino acids, fatty acids, peptides, prostaglandins, purines, catecholamines, and indole alkylamines, as modulators of synaptic and neuronal excitability. Some idea of the scope of the problem ahead is that over two dozen agents are now suspected of exerting powerful effects on neuronal activity, many of which appear to operate through cyclic nucleotides to modify protein synthesis, receptor distribution, and function. What is more intriguing is the suspicion that some peptides such as vasopressin, which have well-defined actions on peripheral target tissues, may be implicated in a number of complex behavioral and regulatory effects by direct action on different neuronal systems of the brain.

Little can be said at present about the developmental features of systems or neurons that utilize or are influenced by these new, putative transmitter or modulatory agents. It is known that the biogenic amine pathways from the brain stem to the forebrain appear quite early in human fetal development, but it is not known what functions these pathways subserve prior to the establishment of classical synaptic relations. It has been suggested that they influence neuronal differentiation and plasticity of neuronal organization.

What can be said with some assurance about cortical dendrites and dendritic spines is that failure of dendritic spine maturation and dendritic development is almost always associated with neurobehavioral disturbances, including intractable seizures, profound mental retardation, and developmental failure.[7] An intriguing recent finding in examining cortical biopsy tissue from infants and young children with developmental failure is that microtubules in dendrites appear geometrically disorganized. In normal cortical neurons, microtubules exhibit parallel conformation in relation to the long axis of dendrites or dendritic branches.

In striking contrast to this, microtubules in dendrites showing early stages of dystrophy or degeneration exhibit whorls, orthogonal relations to each other, and frank dissarray.[8] Since microtubules are components of the cytoskeletal system of neurons, and presumably play a role in the transport of metabolic constituents from neuron cell body out to dendritic terminals, and vice versa, it is likely that perturbations of microtubule orientation secondary to different metabolic insults may be a critical factor in the onset of dendritic and dendritic spine alterations common to a number of developmental disturbances of infancy and childhood associated with mental retardation and developmental failure.

The fact that much of the synaptic organization of the human cerebrum is well-defined in the newborn infant suggests that the potential functional capacity of the normal neonate's information processing systems is considerably greater than has heretofore been appreciated. Since the *density* of synapses in frontal cortex of the normal human neonate is similar to that of the young adult,[9] there is nothing immature about the neuropil of the newborn's cerebral cortex. This is not the case for the output elements of neurons, the axons, which generally undergo myelination over a variable period postnatally, depending in part on neuronal typology.

Developmental neurobiology has unearthed a complex metabolic signaling system between neurons and myelin-forming glial cells. Evidently the system is subject to a host of hormonal metabolic and genetic derangements of infancy and early childhood that lead to dysmyelination or hypomyelination, and ultimately to disturbance or failure of impulse initiation and conduction in myelinated pathways.

Leaving aside further consideration of factors that affect the sequential maturation of neuronal organizations and their projection systems, it is instructive to note several additional areas of neurobiological inquiry that intersect with problems of developmental medicine. One such area is represented by the lysosomal hydrolase deficiency disorders, such as the gangliosidoses, which generally lead to progressive neurobehavioral deterioration. Until recently the onset of neurological and behavioral disturbances in ganglioside storage disease has been attributed to progressive accumulation and cytotoxic action of incomplete products of glycolipid metabolism in swollen neurons.

Alternative views presented in the past few years derive from observations of the geometric features of neurons in human and feline ganglioside storage diseases.[10] Such studies have revealed that neurons laden with membranous cytoplasmic bodies—the pathognomonic cytosome of several of the gangliosides—have acquired new structural compartments studded with dendritic-like spines. In addition, such giant structures, designated meganeurites, frequently give rise to secondary neurites that may differentiate into aberrant dendritic systems.[11] In a word, neuron storage disease is much more than *storage* disease! For it appears that accumulation of lipid catabolites, secondary to lysosomal hydrolase deficiency, turns on the machinery for synthesis and insertion of new surface membrane, including postsynaptic spine receptor elements, into aberrant structural sites. Evidently accumulation per se of membranous cytoplasmic bodies in swollen neurons in feline ganglioside storage disease does not affect the normal electrogenic properties or the synaptic activities of swollen neurons.[12]

These observations identify the lipid storage diseases and related disorders of infancy and childhood as a subject area of interaction between developmental neurobiology and academic pediatrics. If attempts are to be made to ameliorate the neurobehavioral signs of glycolipid accumulation in the brain by enzyme replacement therapy it behooves the investigator in developmental medicine to acquire familiarity with accumulating data on the developmental pathobiology of neurons.[13]

The revolution effected by the discovery of sensitive radioimmunoassay techniques, methods for detecting cell surface antigens, and the use of monoclonal antibodies, as well as refined cell culture systems, has had a major impact on developmental neurobiology. Studies of dissociated cell systems and mechanisms of reaggregation and neuronal differentiation have added new dimensions to in vitro investigations of synapse and receptor development and turnover.

Hypothalamic cell culture systems are currently in use to study the ontogenesis of steroid receptor expression, a problem that bears on the study of sexual dimorphism in the brain and on the field of reproductive biology. It is but a matter of time until many of the steroid and peptide receptors of limbic forebrain neuronal organizations involved in regulatory hypothalamic-hypophyseal and autonomic-adrenomedullary functions will be characterized, particularly from a developmental standpoint.

Neuronal differentiation involves both new process formation and in some instances resorbtion of processes characteristic of earlier fetal stages of development. Genetic metabolic disturbances commonly interdict or retard the growth and development of neurites, since for the overwhelming majority of neurons absorption of primitive cell processes is not a cardinal feature of the developmental program.

One class of neurons, the Purkinje cells of the cerebellum, is unique in exhibiting prominent perisomatic protoplasmic processes (pseudodendrites) in early fetal stages. In the human cerebellum such perisomatic processes are absorbed by the thirty-fifth week of gestation, at which time the soma of the Purkinje cell exhibits a smooth contour interrupted at the apex of the cell by the primary dendrite.[14] It is of interest that in Menkes' disease—X-chromosome-linked copper malabsorption syndrome—there is a failure of perisomatic process reabsorption. The so-called "somatic sprouts" in this condition are polydendrite processes with dendritic spines.[15]

It is suggested that in this genetic metabolic disorder of copper metabolism, oxidative enzyme deficiencies result in failure of the soma membrane of the Purkinje cell to reorganize, which causes retention and aberrant growth of the dendritic structures and dendritic spine membrane. It is curious that failure of cell body differentiation of Purkinje cells, that is, the loss of fetal perisomatic processes, also occurs in association with multiple cardiac anomalies[16] and renal cystic diseases.[17] Are there histogenetic markers common to Purkinje cells and heart and renal cell systems?

The foregoing brief account of several developmental neurobiological problem areas that bear on academic pediatrics raises the question: How much should the academic pediatrician know about neurobiology, and when should she/he learn about it? Surely data indicative of the maturational status of cortical neurons at different antenatal and postnatal stages should be known to all perinatologists. Furthermore the fact that maturational changes in cortical morphology are paralled by distinctive alterations in the electrographic characteristics of visual evoked responses in the preterm infant should certainly be of interest as an objective measure of overt brain function in the face of impending crises.[18,19]

The academic pediatrician should also be aware of advances made in the past decade in the study of different excitable membranes, including alterations in the electrogenic properties of neurons during ontogenesis. It is evident that the classic Hodgkin-Huxley formulations concerning voltage-dependent, sodium-potassium permeability changes underlying the nerve impulse are by no means complete descriptions; nor for that matter were they meant to be. A number of additional voltage-sensitive conductances, some involving calcium as well as sodium and potassium, have now been described. Of particular relevance is the observation that immature neurons may generate action potentials and graded responses due to changes in voltage-dependent calcium permeability.[20] Calcium spikes rather than sodium may dominate the electrogenesis of dendrites of such neurons even in the mature state. These data emphasize the importance of mechanisms regulating calcium metabolism in the immature brain. They point to the critical role of calcium, not only in transmitter release processes, but in the functional activity of dendrites and growing neurites of neurons in active states of process differentiation.[21]

A current subject area of intense interest in neurobiological circles, and one of obvious importance to pediatrics, is that concerned with "neuronal plasticity." Several issues here are frequently confounded in the polemics of "specificity versus plasticity" and in questions bearing on the modifiability of the brain. That the brain is functionally modifiable is self-evident from even a casual consideration of the strategies underlying cognitive development in infancy and childhood.

There is now good evidence from the visual system in subhuman primates for an early period of plasticity in the establishment of the functional and structural integrity of neuronal pathways involved in binocular interaction.[22] Up to a certain period postnatally, perhaps three months, an imbalance in visual input produced by a variety of maneuvers, ranging from monocular occlusion to orbital torsion, results in significant morphophysiological changes in neurons at subcortical and cortical sites. Evidently the monkey's visual system undergoes hard-wiring after this critical period, and thereafter is no longer significantly modifiable by sensory deprivation.

Early monocular visual deprivation produces profound deficits in binocularly driven neurons of visual cortex: reverse suture prior to the end of the critical period leads to reactivation of cortical synaptic pathways driven by the previously deprived eye. This is indicative of a remarkable degree of modifiability of initially genetically programmed neuronal circuitry in the primate brain in the early postnatal period. Since the elegant pioneering studies of D. H. Hubel and T. N. Wiesel,[23] many studies have demonstrated varying degrees of modifiability of developing as well as some mature neuronal systems in the mammalian brain and spinal cord.[24]

There is firm evidence for the capacity of intact neural pathways to sprout collaterals and occupy synaptic sites vacated by the loss of the original "correct" projections,[25] and in some instances recovery of function lost by the initial lesion. There is the alternative possibility, however, that the "rewiring" of synaptic organizations secondary to collateral sprouting after damage to a particular system may also yield *aberrant behaviors!*[26]

The study of "brain plasticity" in developmental neurobiology has been greatly facilitated by the discovery of a number of nerve growth-promoting factors isolated from different tissues. While it appears at the present writing that these trophic factors are of limited efficacy in the mammalian brain, the search for endogenous growth-promoting substances continues unabated. What determines the capacity of some types of neuronal systems, such as those rich in biogenic amines, to sprout new collaterals following damage, even in the mature brain,[27] while other neuronal systems are devoid of this property, remains to be clarified.

It is certain, however, that future advances in the biology of neuronal growth regulation will greatly influence developmental medicine, particularly in the management of the brain-damaged infant. Apropos of this, the past year has witnessed the feasibility of lower mammals restoring the biochemical and functional properties of basal ganglia regions rendered deficient in dopamine projections by grafting implants of midbrain structures from donor animals.[28] Reinnervation of other damaged brain areas such as the hippocampus by axons arising from embryonic implants has also been observed.

While the notion of "brain-grafting" seems like so much sci-fi in respect to the therapeutic management of brain damage, a considerable amount of money, effort, and talent is being expended by the National Institutes of Health and other health agencies throughout the world in pursuit of this fantasy. It remains an open question whether clinical application of these remarkable laboratory findings will be seriously entertained— at least for the next six months!

If there is a take-home message from the present narrative it probably should be an affirmation of the unbridled enthusiasm and energy that characterize the present state of the science dedicated to the pursuit of brain-behavior mechanisms.

As with each passing year the intellectual and technological accomplishments draw the neurobiologist closer to unraveling the secrets of nervous system operations, the spinoff of knowledge relevant to academic pediatrics will surely increase continuously. In the final analysis it is the pediatrician who is charged with the health maintenance of the "competent child." And since "competency" implies a normally functioning brain there is every reason to encourage a growing liaison between the developmental neurobiologist and the pediatrician to achieve this objective. The outcome of this happy union may well be the creation of a new field of *developmental neuromedicine* in which the special skills of the academic pediatrician and the neuroscientist are brought to bear on regulatory problems in child development. If academic pediatrics is in need of a spiritual uplift it might well benefit from a voyage through the foramen magnum and communion with the acme of the biological evolution: the brain.

NOTES

1. *Report of the Task Force on Basic Science to the National Advisory Neurological and Communicative Disorders and Stroke Council,* Chairman, D. P. Purpura, NIH Publication #79-1920 (Bethesda, Maryland: National Institutes of Health, 1979).

2. M. E. Molliver, I. Kostović, and H. Van Der Loos, "The Development of Synapses in Cerebral Cortex of the Human Fetus," *Brain Research* 50 (1970): 403–07.

3. R. Sidman and P. Rakic, "Neuronal Migration with Special Reference to Developing Human Brain: A Review," *Brain Research* 66 (1973): 1–36.

4. N. Zecevic and P. Rakic, "Differentiation of Purkinje Cells and Their Relationship to Other Components of Developing Cerebellar Cortex in Man," *Journal of Comparative Neurology* 167 (1976): 27–47.

5. D. P. Purpura, "Morphogenesis of Visual Cortex in the Preterm Infant," in *Growth and Development of the Brain,* ed. M. A. B. Brazier (New York: Raven Press, 1975): 33–40.

6. ———, "Structure-Dysfunction Relations in the Visual Cortex of Preterm Infants," in *Brain Dysfunction in Infantile Febrile Convulsions,* ed. M. A. B. Brazier and F. Coceani (New York: Raven Press, 1976): 223–40.

7. ———, "Dendritic Differentiation in Human Cerebral Cortex: Normal and Aberrant Developmental Patterns," in *Advances in Neurology,* vol. 12, ed. G. W. Kreutzberg (New York: Raven Press, 1975): 91–116.

8. D. P. Purpura, K. Suzuki, I. Rapin, et al., "Dendritic Varicosities and Microtubule Disarray in Human Cortical Neurons in Developmental Failure," *Proceedings of the Society for Neuroscience,* in press.

9. P. R. Huttenlocher, "Synaptic Density in Human Frontal Cortex—Developmental Changes and Effects of Aging," *Brain Research* 163 (1979): 195–205.

10. D. P. Purpura and K. Suzuki, "Distortion of Neuronal Geometry and Formation of Aberrant Synapses in Neuronal Storage Disease," *Brain Research* 116 (1976): 1–21.

11. D. P. Purpura, "Ectopic Dendritic Growth in Mature Pyramidal Neurons in Human Ganglioside Storage Disease," *Nature* 276 (1978): 520–21.

12. D. P. Purpura, S. M. Highstein, A. B. Karabelas, et al., "Intracellular Recording and HRP-Staining of Cortical Neurons in Feline Ganglioside Storage Disease," *Brain Research* 181 (1980): 446–49.

13. D. P. Purpura, "Pathobiology of Cortical Neurons in Metabolic and Unclassified Amentias," in *Congenital and Acquired Cognitive Disorders,* ed. R. Katzman (New York: Raven Press, 1979): 43–68.

14. Zecevic and Rakic, "Differentiation of Purkinje Cells" (See note 4).

15. D. P. Purpura, A. Hirano, and J. H. French, "Polydendritic Purkinje Cells in X-Chromosome-Linked Copper Malabsorption: A Golgi Study," *Brain Research* 117 (1976): 125–29.

16. Purpura, "Pathobiology of Cortical Neurons" (See note 13).

17. S. Kornguth, L. Knobeloch, C. Viseskul, et al., "Defect of Cerebellar Purkinje Cell Histogenesis Associated with Type I and Type II Renal Cystic Disease," *Acta Neuropathologica* (Berlin) 40 (1977): 1–9.

18. Purpura, "Morphogenesis of Visual Cortex" (See note 5).

19. ———, "Structure-Dysfunction Relations" (See note 6).

20. R. Llinas and M. Sugimori, "Calcium Conductances in Purkinje Cell Dendrites; Their Role in Development and Integration," *Progress in Brain Research* 15 (1979): 323–34.

21. Ibid.

22. S. LeVay, T. N. Wiesel, and D. H. Hubel, "The Development of Ocular Dominance Columns in Normal and Visually Deprived Monkeys," *Journal of Comparative Neurology* 191 (1980): 1–52.

23. Ibid.

24. C. Cotman, ed., *Neuronal Plasticity* (New York: Raven Press, 1978): 325.

25. G. Raisman, "Neuronal Plasticity in the Septal Nuclei of the Adult Rat," *Brain Research* 14 (1969): 25–48.

26. Cotman, *Neuronal Plasticity* (See note 24).

27. A. Björklund and U. Stenevi, "Regeneration of Monoaminergic and Cholinergic Neurons in the Mammalian Central Nervous System," *Physiological Reviews* 59 (1979): 62–100.

28. A. Björklund, "Formation of Connections by Intracerebral Neural Transplants: Specificity and Recovery of Function" (Paper presented at the First Meeting of the International Society for Developmental Neuroscience, Strasbourg, 1980): L13, pp. 32–33.

SCHOOLS OF PUBLIC HEALTH AND ACADEMIC PEDIATRICS

Bernard G. Greenberg,
Frank A. Loda,
*and Earl Siegel**

INTRODUCTION

The current status and the future of academic pediatrics as they relate to schools of public health raise issues and relationships relevant to the deliberations of this conference. In considering these relationships it is well to know something of the history of American schools of medicine and of public health because of their close linkages and comparable lines of development during the first half of this century.

Such a history probably should start with the publication of the Flexner report in 1910,[1] in which the Medical Department of the Johns Hopkins University was cited as the prototype model.† An interesting feature of this developmental period is that the four oldest medical schools were located in private institutions; the growth of such non-tax-supported schools accelerated after the Flexner report was issued. It was not until

---

* Dr. Loda is professor and chief, Division of Community Pediatrics, School of Medicine, and lecturer, Department of Maternal and Child Health, School of Public Health; Dr. Siegel is clinical professor, Department of Pediatrics, School of Medicine, and professor, Department of Maternal and Child Health, School of Public Health, University of North Carolina. Only Dean Greenberg attended the conference.

† A brief history of medical schools before that era may be found in the book by Vernon W. Lippard,[2] especially in the notes at the end of the first chapter.

after World War II that medical schools affiliated with state and municipal universities started to emerge in large numbers.

A similar line of development occurred among schools of public health located in private institutions. Formal instruction in public health in the United States started in the private medical schools because of their interests in bacteriology and sanitation. Some offered formal academic degrees or certificates equivalent to a degree in public health.

The first school of public health was established in 1913 as the Harvard–Massachusetts Institute of Technology School for Health Officers. It closed after only nine years, however, because the courts of Massachusetts ruled that the charters of the two institutions did not permit the granting of a joint degree.

In the meantime, in 1914 the Rockefeller Foundation commissioned William Henry Welch and Wickliffe Rose to formulate a plan for a training program for health personnel that would be an integral part of a university and its medical school. The Welch-Rose report, completed in 1915 and published in the foundation's 1916 *Annual Report,* had an effect similar to that of the Flexner report. It recommended that institutes of hygiene "would not only train health officers but would react upon the medical school of the university and contribute to the training of physicians going into general practice."[3]

Thus the basic design for schools of public health incorporated the education of medical students. The Johns Hopkins University was the first institution to implement the Welch-Rose report; its Institute of Hygiene and Public Health was founded in 1916, with Welch as its director, with a grant from the General Education Board of the Rockefeller Foundation. It opened its doors in 1918.

In 1922 the reorganized Harvard School of Public Health, following the Hopkins pattern, moved off on its own. At that time the private educational institutions were predominant in the field, and the medical schools of Yale, Columbia, and Tulane universities soon created departments of public health; in that respect they differed from the Hopkins and Harvard models of separate schools.

The stimulus for schools of public health in state universities started earlier than the growth of state-financed medical schools. The Social Security Act of 1935 and the amendments of 1936 contained clauses calling for the continuing education of public health personnel. The call was answered by states such as North Carolina and Minnesota, where new schools of public health were soon located in state universities. Michigan already had a public health program in its medical school, and in 1944 it became an independent school of public health. Despite the location of public health programs in state universities, all, or almost all, of the funding came from the federal government.

After World War II schools of public health in state universities began to receive state funds for their support. As a result a primary mission of these schools was to train personnel to work in local and state departments of health. This drifting away from close association with the medical schools and the training of medical students was an abandonment of one of the goals envisioned in the Welch-Rose report. By 1962 there were twelve schools of public health, half of them private and half in tax-supported institutions; since then, nine additional schools have been accredited, all of them state-supported. For a listing of the twenty-one schools see the appendix to this chapter.

While schools of public health were drifting away from the medical schools, the latter in turn were concentrating on biomedical research, with diminished interest in community health problems. Even the new state medical schools derived most of their support from the National Institutes of Health and other granting agencies that promoted biomedical research and training.

A combination of several factors has helped to reunite the interests of the two types of professional schools. In the early to mid-1960s the Great Society movement had an impact on all universities, especially on schools of medicine. This has been documented in excellent detail by E. Riska and others.[4] The movement resulted in a renewed interest in the community, and as a result medical schools began to develop departments of community medicine and family medicine; some departments of pediatrics established divisions of community pediatrics.

The 1977 report of the Task Force on Pediatric Education was a singularly important study of the interface of academic pediatrics and schools of public health.[5] It recommended a substantial expansion of educational experiences at the undergraduate and residency levels, focusing on the biosocial factors that affect the health status and health care of children. The failure of the infant mortality rate to decline and the burgeoning juvenile problems in the late 1960s were added incentives for academic pediatrics to look beyond biomedical and physical factors in the environment.

Coming from the other direction was the report of the Milbank Memorial Fund Commission, *Higher Education for Public Health*,[6] which tended to summarize the misgivings many faculty members in schools of public health were expressing about the failure of their institutions to participate in community health affairs. The report drew attention to the need to study the entire health care delivery system, especially access to and utilization of primary care. The major role of pediatrics in primary care was stressed, as was the need for maternal and child health academic faculty to look beyond their own walls. The report also emphasized the need for heavy reliance on the specialized methods of epidemiology and biostatistics, management sciences, social policy, and the social and behavioral sciences. Thus schools of public health were redirected back toward the providers of health care, and their maternal and child health faculty were urged to develop closer relationships with departments of pediatrics to carry out their own public health missions.

The two types of schools were therefore motivated by several forces to turn toward one another. From the standpoint of pediatrics, the resources to study biosocial factors, the community, and the risk factors associated with primary prevention were heavily concentrated in schools of public health. Clearly the priorities of pediatrics coincided with the mission and academic programs of schools of public health.

As academic pediatrics looks at the 1980s and beyond an even higher priority must be given to studies of human development, preventive medicine, and health care services for all children. It is therefore germane to ask how well academic departments of pediatrics interact with schools of public health, and vice versa.

METHOD OF STUDY

To ascertain the present relationship of schools of public health and academic departments of pediatrics, the authors proceeded in two stages. As a first step they made a thorough review of the University of North Carolina experience. The School of Public Health has a department of Maternal and Child Health (MCH), and the Department of Pediatrics of the School of Medicine has a Division of Community Pediatrics. These and other units in both settings were studied after an extensive review of areas of potential collaboration. Information was obtained regarding teaching at the student, house staff, and postresidency levels in the medical school; research, service, and continuing education were the categories of non-curricular activities covered.

We reviewed the School of Public Health's educational, research, and consultative activities within the School of Medicine and the North Carolina Memorial Hospital, and separated out those related to the Department of Pediatrics. It is clear that many personnel in pediatrics interact with faculty in epidemiology and biostatistics, although the major lines of communication are through MCH. Similarly, personnel in the School of Public Health have contacts with pediatrics through the Robert Wood Johnson Clinical Scholars Program and other groups outside the context of the Department of Pediatrics itself.

Nevertheless the primary efforts are between MCH and pediatrics. One clear observation made was that collaboration is at the postdoctoral level in teaching, research, and service. The MCH faculty do not directly influence the clinical training of medical students as envisioned sixty-five years ago by Welch and Rose, but they are perhaps doing so indirectly by their impact on the pediatric faculty who teach medical students. Faculty in departments in the School of Public Health, such as biostatistics, epidemiology, and parasitology, teach undergraduate medical students in the preclinical years.

Because it was thought that this large number of local collaborative research efforts might be unique to the University of North Carolina, the second stage of our investigation examined patterns elsewhere. Of the twenty-one accredited schools of public health, a sample of nine was selected for detailed study* because they are large, well-established, and affiliated with a school of medicine. The respondents were the deans and/or professors of MCH, who were deemed to be the most knowledgeable about the interrelationships between academic pediatrics and their respective schools. Telephone conversations were followed by a structured questionnaire soliciting specific written responses. Only one of the nine failed to respond in writing. To supplement the reports, a member of the pediatrics departments in about half the affiliated medical schools was contacted.

To better assess the role in and value of a school of public health to a department of pediatrics, the authors identified a sample of eight departments of pediatrics in medical schools with no school of public health on the site.† Two of these departments are in medical schools that award the equivalent of a master of public health degree, and thus considerable public health knowledge, skills, and activities exist. The methods of contact were in general the same as in the sample of schools of public health, namely, a telephone call followed by a questionnaire.

As with the schools of public health, the eight departments of pediatrics did not constitute a scientifically designed random sample; they were selected because it was believed or known that the faculty and students are active in community services. The authors therefore do not suggest that the data are rep-

---

* University of California at Berkeley, University of California at Los Angeles, Columbia University, Johns Hopkins University, University of Minnesota, University of North Carolina, University of Texas at Houston, University of Washington, and Yale University.

† University of Arizona, Baylor University, Boston University (which has now established a School of Public Health for which it is seeking accreditation), McGill University, University of Pennsylvania, University of Rochester, University of Southern California, and University of Texas, Galveston Branch.

resentative of all medical schools or all schools of public health. The samples do, however, provide an instructive picture of what is happening in some of the large schools of public health and in some community-oriented departments of pediatrics.

Schools of Public Health

Slightly different information was requested from the institutional groups. The *schools of public health* were asked for the following information:

• Types of faculty and trainees involved in exchanges between the department of pediatrics and the school of public health, and what such exchanges involve in terms of teaching, research, service, continuing education, and technical assistance.

• The role of "third party" centers and institutes in fostering interactions, as well as that of special training activities such as the Johnson Clinical Scholars Program.

• The role of a specific division, particularly ambulatory or community pediatrics, as a focus of interaction.

• The impact of trends in societal needs and demands for health care, as well as trends in pediatric education.

• The function of public and private funding in fostering collaboration.

• The areas of primary concern that stimulate increased interaction.

• The limitations on exchanges of services and personnel, especially institutional factors.

• The extent to which interaction is dependent on certain individuals.

• An assessment of future relationships of departments of pediatrics and schools of public health.

Departments of Pediatrics

The *departments of pediatrics* were asked to respond to the following:

• The effect of the absence of a school of public health on the development of departmental programs, especially in general pediatrics, ambulatory pediatrics, and community pediatrics.

• The use of departmental faculty to provide knowledge and skills typically associated with a school of public health, in, for example, epidemiology, biostatistics, and MCH.

• The roles of community medicine, preventive medicine, or similar departments in filling these needs.

• Any ties that may exist with a geographically separate school of public health.

• The perceived priority attached by the respondent and her/his institution to having an affiliated school of public health.

In light of the demand made upon the respondents, the details provided were varied. Nevertheless the cooperation was almost complete, and the authors are indeed grateful to the individuals who provided the information.

RESULTS

It is clear that the presence of a school of public health and a department of pediatrics at the same university does not assure a productive interchange. Two of the schools of public health reported there are practically no areas of collaboration with the medical school's pediatric faculty. It should be noted, however, that one of these schools is geographically separated from the medical school by a matter of forty-five to sixty min utes of travel time. The other indicated there is little receptivity on the part of the department of pediatrics to the specialized educational and research expertise residing in the school of public health; in an attempt to ascertain how the faculty in pediatrics at that university perceive the interaction, it was later learned there was a modicum of exchange.

The teaching of pediatrics to undergraduate medical students by public health faculty received little mention, but some pediatric faculty indicated participation in the teaching programs of schools of public health. An important factor in public health input to the medical school relates to the Johnson Clinical Scholars Programs. The capacity to attract and to retain funding for these programs seems highly correlated with the presence of a school of public health and its active relationship with the department of pediatrics.

One area of major interaction is support of education and research activities in ambulatory pediatric residency and fellowships programs. Illustrative of the large variety of substantive pediatric problems involved in joint teaching and research are perinatal epidemiology; child abuse and neglect; sudden infant death syndrome; genetics; psychosocial factors in family relationships; adolescent health; and international health.

The unique strengths that schools of public health are able to bring to academic departments of pediatrics were consistently emphasized by the respondents; research design, specific research methods, data management, and data analyses were mentioned repeatedly. Motivation to take advantage of these strengths is influenced by shifts in societal and medical education priorities.

This was referred to earlier as an effect of the Great Society movement that began in the mid-1960s. Increasing emphasis on primary care and the provision of health services led to the recognition that rigorous research methods must be applied to these two aspects of medical care. Externally funded programs such as the Johnson Clinical Scholars Program, health services research projects, and large adolescent health research grants were cited by respondents as playing important roles in stimulating such research.

Interactions were initially dependent on certain personalities, but this was viewed as the usual way in which interdepartmental or interschool cooperation begins. Once the relationships are established, however, they appear to be mutually valued and their future is characterized by such expressions as "closer," "bright," "essential," and "enthusiastic." Concern was expressed about continuing funding, constraints on faculty time, and administrative support from deans and departmental heads.

Chapel Hill as an Example

A few comments concerning the Chapel Hill situation may amplify the general picture. In an initial detailed review we found a number of meaningful interactions encompassing such areas as joint faculty appointments; faculty development activities; the Johnson Clinical Scholars Program; the general preventive medicine residency program; specific course participation; joint MCH/community pediatrics seminar series; and clinical teaching in the outpatient department and the newborn nursery.

Collaborative research includes evaluative studies in primary care, rural health, and child health services in local health departments; a controlled evaluation of regional perinatal care; genetics; child abuse and neglect; environmental factors in childhood respiratory diseases; effects of family ritual on illness; and the pediatrician's impact on parent-infant behavior through well-child visits.

These interactions at Chapel Hill, particularly as they relate to research activities, tend to be reciprocally supportive, making it difficult to assign to the contributions a predominant direction from either the School of Public Health or the Department of Pediatrics.

Moreover there has been an increasing level of interaction with the School of Public Health on the part of pediatric residents interested in preventive medicine and public health, as well as postresidency trainees such as Johnson Clinical Scholars and pediatric faculty members. About half the Clinical Scholars in Chapel Hill obtain an M.P.H. degree with specialization in epidemiology or MCH. Even those medical students and pediatric residents with no special interest in community health are indirectly exposed to content, attitudes, and skills by the School of Public Health through faculty and trainees in the Department of Pediatrics who have considerable involvement with the school.

Along with most of the respondents we observe a major facilitation of relationships through "third parties" such as the University of North Carolina Child Development Institute, the Health Services Research Center, the general preventive medicine residency program, and the repeatedly emphasized Johnson Clinical Scholars Program.

Finally, an essential ingredient is a critical mass of faculty in both the Department of Pediatrics and the School of Public

Health who attach high value to the relationships. The creation of the Division of Community Pediatrics at Chapel Hill about a decade ago became a focal point to facilitate communication between the Department of Pediatrics and the School of Public Health. Support by the chairman of the department is strong and visible, and he, along with two other faculty members, spent sabbatical years at the School of Public Health, thus reflecting the level of priority assigned to the relationship.

As for faculty in MCH, several members, including the third author, have a long-standing commitment to strengthening the partnership between the clinical departments in the School of Medicine and the School of Public Health in order to enhance their effectiveness. The deans of the two schools have also helped to foster a close working relationship during the past decade.

Departments Not Affiliated with Public Health Schools

When one considers pediatrics departments in universities that do not have schools of public health, the first question that comes to mind is: Do these departments have less strength in community pediatrics?

The results clearly confirm the authors' judgment in picking departments of pediatrics that have excellent community programs. There is no evidence that these programs are stronger in universities with schools of public health than in the eight selected departments.

This is not to say that, in the absence of a school of public health, pediatrics departments do not need the intellectual resources available in the schools, such as epidemiology, biostatistics, and MCH. In fact the impressive thing about those departments with strong programs in community pediatrics is that they are systematically helping to develop such resources in the medical school. The programs are most often based in a department of preventive or community medicine, with heavy emphasis on biostatistics, epidemiology, and community programs. In a few schools many of these resources are placed in the pediatrics department itself. In the remaining schools the resources are housed in a variety of locations—including the dean's office. The important thing is that the body of knowledge that is classically associated with a school of public health is incorporated, almost without exception, with programs that emphasize ambulatory pediatrics. This suggests that these resources are essential for effective programs of community pediatrics.

Many medical schools that have active community pediatrics programs in association with other departments or programs also tend to develop a M.P.H. degree program or an equivalent master's program. Having graduate students train in areas such as epidemiology, health administration, and biostatistics appears important to a well-developed program.

The question naturally arises as to whether these M.P.H. degree programs are the equivalent of those provided in an accredited school of public health, which may have deeper strengths in the three disciplines mentioned and a wider breadth of coverage in the social and behavioral sciences. Putting aside the question of accreditation for these degrees, it appears that those medical schools that have developed strong ambulatory and community pediatrics programs have done so because of forceful leadership in the pediatrics department. It requires a major commitment by politically influential leadership in the medical school to achieve what has been accomplished in such universities in the absence of a public health school. Fortunately, there are a number of such leaders in academic pediatrics.

The next issue that emerges is whether the programs established by the medical schools are in fact stronger than those that depend on a relationship between a school of medicine and a school of public health. A few of the respondents did indeed suggest they enjoy a closer relationship with their colleagues because they are in the same medical school rather than in a separate school of public health. They claim the administrative arrangements allow the groups to work together more closely, with less parochialism interfering with their collaboration. This may be a rationalization in the absence of an experiment or trial to compare the two possible arrangements, but programs in schools of medicine, particularly those in departments of pediatrics, clearly tend to be more directly responsive to the specific goals of that department. The question of whether this is desirable must remain unanswered at this time. Respondents in a school of public health might argue that breadth of vision is sacrificed to advance more parochial interests.

Quality of Programs in Medical Schools
Not Affiliated with Public Health Schools

This brings up the next question of whether programs in a school of medicine can develop the depth of resources available in a school of public health. There certainly is a tendency for the lone epidemiologist, or the small group of epidemiologists, in a department of community medicine or pediatrics to be overworked and intellectually isolated. It also appears logical that epidemiologists, for example, are more productive in their specific area when they are associated with faculty in their own and other disciplines in a school of public health. We did not attempt to collect data on this point.

An increasing number of departments of pediatrics are recruiting faculty who have formal training in public health disciplines. Such departments point to these individuals as examples of their dedication to community pediatrics and public health issues. It remains to be seen how well these faculty members function over time unless they are supported and/or challenged by colleagues with similar interests.

As mentioned earlier, the increased emphasis in recent years on programs such as the Johnson Clinical Scholars Program and interdisciplinary institutes has promoted interest in community pediatrics programs. The general pediatrics training programs sponsored by the Johnson Foundation have the potential to create another focus around which groups of scholars in both types of schools can develop. These programs promote active collaboration between schools of medicine and schools of public health, but a serious problem may arise when extramural funding shrinks or ceases. The long-term institutionalization of such programs may be in jeopardy, and that may in turn jeopardize some of the active collaboration of the two schools.

The issue was raised in the questionnaire of the desirability of a university that does not have a school of public health establishing one. In an era of increasing fiscal problems one might think they would be reluctant to consider the development of a major new school. As indicated earlier, however, Boston University has since opened a School of Public Health; the others do not consider it a priority item. We are aware of three other new schools of public health that are in the process of being established, and state commissions in Florida, New York, and New Jersey, for example, have been appointed to consider the issue. Whether or not a decision is made to go ahead, the data suggest that for those universities with no affiliated school of public health it appears essential that other institutional structures be created so that academicians concerned about social pediatrics have an environment that will stimulate their intellectual development and act as a spur to establish a comprehensive curriculum in community pediatrics.

DISCUSSION

Since the beginning of the present century pediatrics has probably been the clinical discipline that has placed the most emphasis on community programs and public health issues. The era of rapidly expanding biomedical research in the 1950s and 1960s, together with increasing pediatric subspecialization, caused many departments to move away from such concerns. Faculty interested in community health and related areas frequently found themselves isolated from the highly technical biomedical research of their own colleagues. Many pediatrics departments established in the twenty-year period after World War II showed a diminished orientation toward traditional pediatric concerns of public health and community medicine. Beginning in the mid-1960s this attitude began to change as pediatrics departments attempted to reintroduce more biosocial and community medicine into their curricula. This development failed to occur to the same degree in departments of medicine, which perhaps contributed to the growth of departments of community medicine and family medicine in the medical schools.

From the results of this small survey it is clear that strong programs in community pediatrics can be developed in the absence of a school of public health. On the other hand, in a few instances the schools of public health have virtually no interaction with the medical schools' departments of pediatrics. Thus one would have to conclude that at the present time, while a school of public health may be helpful, it is neither necessary nor sufficient for the development of an effective program in community pediatrics in the medical school.

Despite this conclusion, one cannot be completely sanguine about the continuation of strong, self-contained programs in community pediatrics in the medical schools. Such programs require the forceful leadership of one or two persons, and a supporting staff in the core disciplines usually found in public health schools. Where the relationship between community pediatrics and a school of public health has been established, it, too, started with strong leadership, but the important difference is that such collaboration eventually became institutionalized. This kind of arrangement may therefore have a better chance of survival, although the influence of third-party interests may also make it dependent on outside sources of funding.

Finally, it is of concern that many young pediatric faculty members with competence in public health disciplines such as epidemiology, biostatistics, and maternal and child health are entering universities with a frail supporting structure to assure their growth in community pediatrics. This structure can be developed in the absence of a school of public health, but it requires significant resources. This situation will pose definite problems in terms of individual career development for many young academic pediatricians. One way to keep their careers topical and the programs vibrant would be to continually strengthen them by periodic exchanges and sabbaticals, as well as the frequent introduction of outstanding visiting scholars from those disciplines usually housed in a school of public health.

NOTES

1. Abraham Flexner, *Medical Education in the United States and Canada. A Report to the Carnegie Foundation for the Advancement of Teaching*, Bulletin No. Four (Boston: D. B. Updike, Merrymount Press, 1910).

2. Vernon W. Lippard, *A Half-Century of American Medical Education, 1920–1970* (New York: Josiah Macy, Jr. Foundation, 1974).

3. William H. Welch and Wickliffe Rose, "Report on an Institute of Hygiene," *Annual Report* (New York: The Rockefeller Foundation, 1916).

4. Elianne Riska, "Social Reform and Reform in Medical Education," in *Medical Education Since 1960: Marching to a Different Drummer,* ed. Andrew W. Hunt and Lewis E. Weeks (East Lansing: Michigan State University and W. K. Kellogg Foundation, 1979).

5. *The Future of Pediatric Education, Report of the Task Force on Pediatric Education* (Evanston, Illinois: Task Force on Pediatric Education, nd [1978?]).

6. *Higher Education for Public Health,* Report of the Milbank Memorial Fund Commission, Cecil G. Sheps, chairman (New York: Milbank Memorial Fund, 1976).

APPENDIX

SCHOOLS OF PUBLIC HEALTH
IN THE UNITED STATES*

Department of Public Health
School of Medicine
University of Alabama
Birmingham, Alabama

School of Public Health
University of California
Berkeley, California

School of Public Health
University of California
Los Angeles, California

School of Public Health
Columbia University
New York, New York

School of Public Health
Harvard University
Boston, Massachusetts

School of Public Health
University of Hawaii
Honolulu, Hawaii

School of Public Health
University of Illinois
Chicago, Illinois

School of Hygiene and
   Public Health
The Johns Hopkins University
Baltimore, Maryland

School of Public Health
Loma Linda University
Loma Linda, California

Division of Public Health
School of Health Sciences
University of Massachusetts
Amherst, Massachusetts

School of Public Health
University of Michigan
Ann Arbor, Michigan

School of Public Health
University of Minnesota
Minneapolis, Minnesota

School of Public Health
The University of North Carolina
Chapel Hill, North Carolina

College of Health
The University of Oklahoma
Oklahoma City, Oklahoma

Graduate School of Public Health
The University of Pittsburgh
Pittsburgh, Pennsylvania

School of Public Health
The University of Puerto Rico
San Juan, Puerto Rico

---

* Three new schools of public health, at Boston University, San Diego State University, and Tufts University, are currently seeking accreditation.

School of Public Health
University of South Carolina
Columbia, South Carolina

School of Public Health and
   Tropical Medicine
Tulane University
New Orleans, Louisiana

School of Public Health
The University of Texas
Houston, Texas

School of Public Health and
   Community Medicine
The University of Washington
Seattle, Washington

Department of Epidemiology and
   Public Health
School of Medicine
Yale University
New Haven, Connecticut

CURRENT RESIDENCY REQUIREMENTS IN PEDIATRICS: THE RELATIONSHIP OF THE ACADEMICIAN AND THE PRACTITIONER

Edwin L. Kendig, Jr.

The first part of my presentation is essentially a summary of the official *"Special Requirements" for Residency Programs in Pediatrics,*[1] which have been approved by the American Board of Pediatrics (ABP), the Executive Board of the American Academy of Pediatrics (AAP), and the Council on Medical Education of the American Medical Association (AMA). A review of this material is necessary in order to pinpoint existing or potential problems. A few observations and comments have been added.

> Residency programs in pediatrics are organized and conducted to provide an advancing educational experience with increasing patient responsibilities over a period of three years. The Residency Review Committee (RRC) designates the various levels of training as Pediatric Levels (PL) 1, 2, and 3.

PL-1 refers to the first full year of accredited basic or core training in pediatrics, which must include at least eight months in general pediatrics; PL-2 refers to the second core year in which increased assumption of responsibility includes supervisory activities; PL-3 refers to the third year, which may be a chief or senior supervisory residency. The integral requirements of the program have not been altered by the recent revisions. An earlier revision, however, did dictate changes. At present the integral requirements are:

• A year of supervisory experience, including at least six months of direct and senior supervisory responsibility in general pediatrics.

• Subspecialty rotations, if offered, of no less than one month's duration.

• The accumulation of no more than six months in any single subspecialty; the total of all such rotations is not to exceed eleven months.

• The equivalent of at least six months' experience in ambulatory pediatrics, with the recommendation that at least a portion of that period consist of continuing care as well as block assignments.

An accredited program may be independent or it may exist in two or more institutions as an affiliated or integrated undertaking; an integrated program is one in which two or more involved institutions have approved programs; an affiliated program is one in which one of the institutions is not approved.

In both the integrated and affiliated programs the strengths of each institution are utilized to promote a satisfactory educational experience for the house officer. The amount of time spent in each institution should be determined by her/his educational needs rather than by the service needs of the institution. The educational objectives must be described, and copies of formal written agreements and contracts must be submitted.

Accredited programs may use the resources of other appropriate but less closely affiliated institutions to supply certain essential or enriching elements in the training of a house officer. Because the affiliate institution is not approved by the RRC, however, periods of house officer rotation in that institution should total no more than three months in each of the three years of training.

In using an affiliated program it is important that the needs of the house officer, and the requirements for meeting those needs, be explicitly stated in a contract or in an exchange of letters:

• The scope of the affiliation.
• Available resources in the affiliate program.
• Duties and responsibilities of the house officer.

• Relationship of the house officer and the staff of both the affiliate and the primary program.

The house officer must be an active participant in the prevailing pattern of instruction and patient care.

STAFF

Of foremost importance in a successful graduate training program is the quality of supervision and evaluation of the clinical work of the house officers.

Both the program director and the faculty must be effective. They should be certified by the ABP or possess suitable equivalent qualifications. Qualified subspecialists should be incorporated in the program, and junior staff appointments—fourth year of training—may be desirable.

Continuity of leadership is important to the integrity of a program. Whenever a change in director occurs the RRC must reevaluate the program. The senior chief—departmental chairman or program director—will be responsible for all educational activities.

The staff should include qualified members of allied health professions, including adequate numbers of qualified pediatric nurses.

NUMBER OF HOUSE OFFICERS

The exact number of house officers is not designated. Consideration should, however, be given to the ratio of faculty to house staff and house staff to patients. It is important that there be sufficient numbers of house officers to promote interaction, thereby enhancing the learning experience.

SCOPE OF TRAINING AND FACILITIES

Residency programs in pediatrics should be designed and organized to prepare physicians for comprehensive care of the pediatric patient—infant, child, and adolescent. This may be accomplished through a continuum of carefully advancing educational experiences and increasing patient care responsibilities. The program should include adequate training in the basic medical sciences and in the clinical, laboratory, public health, and community aspects of pediatrics.

The resident should have experience with the health supervision of the well child, and should be exposed to diseases encountered in office-based practice; psychological and social issues; and problems in both surgical and medical subspecialty areas; and have experience with minor illnesses, emergency conditions, and chronic illnesses.

Inpatient and outpatient facilities must be adequate in size, variety, and equipment.

AMBULATORY SERVICES

A high quality of ambulatory pediatric care is essential to adequate training.

Pediatric problems of variety and complexity should be represented in the patient care group. Continuity must be established between inpatient and ambulatory services. Certain aspects of ambulatory care deserve special mention:

Continuity (Follow-up) Clinic

Each house officer should have a weekly or biweekly assignment to the clinic, during which she/he is relieved of other duties. Patients should include well children of various ages and those with chronic, often multiple, illnesses. Subspecialty consultants should be available. The house officer should serve in the continuity clinic for at least two years.

Acute Illness Clinic and Emergency Room

This rotation must be adequately supervised and the patient load should be reasonable. The duration of this assignment should be a minimum of three months. Training in minor surgery and orthopedics should be included.

Specialty Clinics

These clinics should provide the house officer with experience as a supervised consultant. Recommendations include experience in dermatology, allergy, neurology, cardiology, psychology, developmental pediatrics, and care of the handicapped and adolescents. Among the other desirable areas of experience are hematology, endocrinology, gastroenterology, pulmonary disorders, renal disease, collagen diseases, and learning problems.

Preceptorships

Office electives for preceptorships may constitute up to two months in either the second or third year. Assignments may be in solid blocks of time or may run concurrent with other assignments. The house officer should be involved in decision making, make hospital visits with the preceptor, and maintain good office records; the house officer should not function merely as an observer. The preceptor should be capable and interested, and must be physically present for the purpose of supervision. The preceptor is responsible for the evaluation of the house officer.

QUANTITATIVE REQUIREMENTS

A numerical quota of patients is not feasible. Programs should have a sufficient number and variety of hospital patients, however, to assure broad training and experience for each house officer. Hospital duties should not be so demanding that a stimulating educational experience is precluded. It is essential that the house officer be taught responsibility for patient care. Night and weekend duty at least every fourth night and weekend is desirable.

BASIC SCIENCE TEACHING

In order to increase the breadth and depth of the educational challenge, participation of basic scientists in clinical rounds and conferences is recommended.

LABORATORY, RADIOLOGY, AND PATHOLOGY FACILITIES

Laboratory, radiology, and pathology services must be available twenty-four hours a day, and must be adequate to allow the house officer to gain an educational experience during the care of patients.

LEARNING EXPERIENCES

The house officer must learn by assuming meaningful responsibility. This may be accomplished by arriving at her/his own diagnostic impressions; by consulting appropriate source materials and persons; and by developing plans for diagnostic studies. The assumption of responsibility must be carefully supervised by the pediatric faculty.

> The most important formal teaching session is attending rounds conducted by a qualified teacher who is immediately available to the house officer for consultation and who is backed by a staff of consultants in specialty areas.

Attendance at other regularly assigned teaching sessions is also necessary.

CONFERENCES

In addition to regular departmental conferences, teaching sessions in pathology, radiology, and the various subspecialties should be conducted. At least once a week there should be a meeting attended by both house staff and teaching staff, and the house officer should be actively involved in that meeting.

CLINICAL INVESTIGATION AND RESEARCH

The opportunity for clinical investigation should be offered, but should not be required.

MEDICAL LIBRARY

An adequate medical library should be available on a twenty-four-hour basis. Access to computerized literature is desirable.

RECORDS

Good records include a careful history and physical examination, study and management plans, progress notes, and summary. A unit record system is recommended for both inpatient and outpatient charts.

EVALUATION

Periodic evaluation of the educational progress of all residents is required.

This can be accomplished by: 1) standard intraining examinations at the beginning of PL-1 and PL-2 years, and, if performance is questionable, at the beginning of the PL-3 years; and 2) inhouse evaluations. These evaluations must be discussed with the resident and kept on file and available for review.

CONCLUSION

A successful program requires time, effort, ability, and enthusiasm on the part of both house officer and faculty.

COMMENT

A pediatric residency now requires three full years in general pediatrics instead of the formerly acceptable combinations, such as two years in general pediatrics and one year in a rotating or mixed internship. Further, it is no longer possible for the candidate to spend two years in general pediatrics and two years in a subspecialty fellowship. Application of this new requirement in regard to subspecialization includes those house officers who were graduated from medical school after 30 June 1978. While not explicitly stated, request for review may be made. Such a review may provide an opportunity for a departmental chairman to arrange the direction of training for a future faculty member.

The recent modification limiting subspecialty rotations to a maximum of six months in any single subspecialty—primarily aimed at reducing the house officer's assignments in the neonatal intensive care unit (ICU)—and the total of such rotations not to exceed eleven months may, however, allow for some differences in interpretation. For example, an institution may assign a PL-2 or PL-3 house officer to the neonatal ICU in a supervisory capacity. Thus this assignment will not be counted as time spent in the neonatal ICU, and patient coverage is provided. This is one interpretation, and it may not be a valid one.*

The present emphasis on primary care has resulted in a two-track system of house staff training. Institutions may opt to provide two completely separate programs, or they may choose to provide the same program for the first two years for those in both tracks, with the program for the third year to be determined when the house officer makes her/his decision in regard to academic work or private practice. Those who choose the academic field will usually spend two or three more years in training, anyway, with perhaps a year as chief resident and two years in subspecialty training.

THE ACADEMICIAN AND THE PEDIATRIC PRACTITIONER

Increased emphasis on ambulatory pediatrics by the ABP, with special attention to psychosocial pediatrics and a program of continuing patient care, reflects a change of philosophy in regard to the practice of pediatrics. In addition, another benefit has been realized, that is, a small but definite improvement in the relationship between pediatricians in the academic setting and those in private practice.

Academicians have historically been largely active in secondary and tertiary patient care. The new direction of pediatrics places more emphasis on primary care. Since private practitioners are almost totally so engaged, their expertise in that area has caused them to be viewed more favorably by the academician. They are therefore being more frequently involved in teaching.

---

* One member of the RRC phrases it thus: "Assignment of the PL-3 trainee to the NICU will be primarily in a supervisory capacity, and should be combined with similar supervisory duties in other areas of responsibility...." This PL-3 trainee must not have major patient care responsibility.

It is clear that an optimal relationship still does not exist, and some changes in the pediatric scene have served to magnify the schism. An example is the regionalization of perinatal care, a movement that has resulted in improved care of the neonate, but that has cost the pediatric practitioner considerable patient responsibility.

What else can be done to improve the relationship between the two groups? In the author's AAP presidential address allusion was made to this problem and *communication* was suggested as the first step toward its solution.[2] Pediatric practitioners could not exist without pediatric teaching programs and research; conversely, the latter would be pragmatically useless without practicing pediatricians. Both groups must recognize that they exist interdependently and that their mutual growth and development is equally interdependent. Understanding between the two groups must begin on the local scene; obviously the level of cooperation and good feeling between academician and practitioner varies from one community to another.

It is my feeling, however, that the AAP possesses the capability and resources to help promote better understanding between these groups. The academy is an organization composed of both practitioners and academicians, and its Executive Board has made and is making every effort to ensure that it represents both groups. The AAP is the *only* organization that represents practitioners, and within the academy there is the Council on Pediatric Practice and the Committee on Practice Management and Ambulatory Medicine; for the academician there is the Committee on Research and the Council on Sections. The Committee on Medical Education serves both groups.

Furthermore, officers of the AAP now meet on a regular basis with officers of the American Pediatric Society, the Society for Pediatric Research, and the Ambulatory Pediatric Association at the time of the AAP annual meeting in the fall and at the annual meetings of the research societies in the spring. These discussions, which deal more often with the support of legislation promoting the health and welfare of children, including pediatric research, constitute efforts to present a unified approach.

Relations between the academician and the practicing

pediatrician are hardly perfect, but they are improving primarily because of the present emphasis on ambulatory pediatrics. Better communication will speed that improvement.

NOTES

1. Liaison Committee on Graduate Medical Education, *"Special Requirements" for Residency Programs in Pediatrics,* Proposed Revisions (np: October 1979).
2. E. L. Kendig, Jr., "Presidential Address: Communication," *Pediatrics* 65 (1980): 622.

DISCUSSANT

Floyd W. Denny

I am concerned about what I interpret as the inflexibility of the requirements outlined by Dr. Kendig for certification by the American Board of Pediatrics.

First, it seems there is the assumption that all pediatric house staff learn and mature at the same rate, an assumption we all know to be far from correct. I agree that the resident who plans to enter the practice of general pediatrics can benefit from three years of general training. Furthermore, it appears there may be enough flexibility in the requirements to allow some of these individuals to get a modest taste of one or two subspecialty areas; I think this is a desirable thing for the appropriate resident.

What concerns me more, however, is the resident who has decided on a career in academic pediatrics and who faces, except in very unusual circumstances, the same restrictions as the resident who plans to enter practice. The number of pediatricians going into clinical research is decreasing drastically; probably one reason for this is the long training period now required to master modern research methods. If an extra clinical year is added, which I think is really unnecessary in many instances, I am afraid we only place another barrier before those interested in an academic career.

I hope very much the board will reconsider the present requirements and reinstitute some of the flexibility that was present in previous requirements.

ACADEMIC PEDIATRICS
IN THE UNITED KINGDOM

O. H. Wolff

ACADEMIC MEDICINE AND
THE NATIONAL HEALTH SERVICE

In order to present a meaningful picture of the present status and future trends of academic pediatrics in the United Kingdom it is necessary first to clarify the relationship of the universities and the National Health Service (NHS) as it affects our teaching hospitals. All academics, including academic pediatricians, are employed by the universities and hold honorary contracts with the NHS. Professors, readers (associate professors), and, in most medical schools, senior lecturers (assistant professors) hold honorary consultant contracts; lecturers (instructors or assistant professors) hold honorary senior registrar contracts. The honorary contract allows them to operate a clinical service, and the senior academic staff carry full clinical responsibility for the patients they see in the hospital.

In most pediatrics departments of teaching hospitals there are, in addition to the academic staff, consultants employed by the NHS, whose appointments may be full time or part time. Part-time consultants in a major specialty such as pediatrics spend most of their working time, about seven to nine half-days, in the teaching hospital. The rest may be spent in another hospital, in research, or in private practice. Consultants in the United Kingdom see private patients only on referral from a family doctor, with the exception of some patients from abroad who may not have a family doctor.

Outside a few large centers, pediatrics does not offer great opportunities for private practice. NHS consultants make an important contribution to the teaching of undergraduates and postgraduates, and they usually hold honorary academic appointments as lecturers or senior lecturers. They have complete clinical independence and the only aspect of their work that is organized by the academics is the teaching program. There are exceptions to this arrangement. In at least one of the thirteen London medical schools the department of pediatrics is staffed entirely by academics; in three of the schools a formal academic department with a professor has not yet been established. As a federal institution, academic developments at the University of London tend to be slower than in the rest of the country. Even in the other universities, however, most academic departments of pediatrics have been established only over the past thirty-five years.

Of the thirty-four medical schools in the United Kingdom, twenty-seven are in England, five in Scotland, and one each in Wales and Northern Ireland. The Institute of Child Health, the medical school of the Hospital for Sick Children, University of London, is devoted chiefly, although not entirely, to postgraduate training in pediatrics. The other thirty-three schools are concerned primarily with undergraduate teaching, but they do make important contributions to postgraduate education. There are no private medical schools in the United Kingdom.

One of the challenges that faces all senior academic pediatricians is how to make the discipline attractive to some of the more promising young doctors; otherwise the future of pediatrics as an academic subject is in danger. It is therefore appropriate for me to try and look with the eyes of the young man or woman who has decided on pediatrics as a career and who now has reached a stage when a decision has to be made about whether to climb the academic ladder or the NHS ladder; fortunately it is not too difficult to move from one across to the other.

Among the advantages of the academic ladder are greater opportunities for research. The NHS consultant may engage in research, but because of the current financial troubles in my country it is unlikely that many consultant appointments with substantial time for research will become available. Moreover it is usually easier for an academic than for a NHS consultant to obtain funds for research. The consultant may also have difficulty in gaining access to laboratories and in finding technical help, except by arrangement with an academic unit. In addition, the consultant is likely to suffer more than the academic from the bureaucratic restrictions and irritations that are common features of work in any large organization such as the NHS, and that tend to become particularly irksome in times of financial difficulty.

The academic has more scope for independent action, especially in terms of obtaining funds for the continuing support of existing ventures and, occasionally, to start new ones. Most academics appreciate this greater independence, which allows them to have visions and work toward them. Unhappily, however, the present financial crisis affects universities as much as it does the NHS, and there is the danger that academic independence may suffer as a result. (I would not wish anyone to conclude from this comparison that I disapprove of the NHS. It is only in detail that I would like to see changes made, and, most important, more money made available to improve the performance of the NHS.)

Financially, the comparison is less favorable for the academic. In theory the basic salary scale for senior academics and consultants is the same, but in practice there exist several minor differences that favor the consultant. To give an example, the NHS undergoes certain administrative changes periodically, and a recent regulation allows full-time consultants to do a limited amount of private practice. Academics are not in general permitted to earn money in private practice, but the fees they do receive make a useful contribution to departmental funds for faculty travel and the purchase of books.

Despite these differences the personal relationships of the academics and the staff of the NHS are usually good, particularly in specialties such as pediatrics, where private practice does not play an important part. Nevertheless, I sometimes wonder whether the atmosphere of the teaching hospital might not benefit if all the senior staff were employed by the university.

FUTURE NEEDS

The primary ambition of most medical school departments is to enlarge the size of their academic staff.[1] Because departments of pediatrics in the United Kingdom were established only relatively recently and in difficult financial times, the number of academic staff is usually inadequate for the clinical, teaching, research, and administrative duties. This deficiency is particularly marked in comparison with departments of longer standing, such as general medicine, surgery, and obstetrics and gynecology. The shortage of staff makes it difficult for the heads of departments to decide where to place the emphasis: on clinical service, teaching, or research.

It is a valued tradition of British medicine for senior staff to continue to provide clinical services. Senior academics, including professors, work in outpatient departments once or twice a week and take full clinical responsibility for patients admitted to the wards under their care. This continuing clinical involvement, although time-consuming, lends reality and depth to their teaching activities. Thus, inevitably, clinical work and teaching take up much of their time.

The main reason more staff is needed is to strengthen our research contribution; but another reason for the limited research output is the shortage of funds. The university budget is not usually sufficient to provide for more than the salaries of the senior academic staff, limited technical assistance, laboratory space, essential equipment, and operating expenses, and it may not even be enough for these basic needs.

Money is allocated to the universities by the University Grants Committee (UGC), which, in turn, receives the funds from the government's Department of Education and Science. The allocation depends on the number of students enrolled rather than on the amount of research being conducted at a university. As for the salaries of younger research workers, the purchase of expensive equipment, and other items, we depend on support from sources outside the university, including the various grant-giving bodies.

Approximately £193 million (US$434.25 million) is available for research in the United Kingdom. Of this sum about £80 million comes from governmental sources—including £50 million from the Medical Research Council (MRC) and £23 million from the Department of Health and Social Security—and £113 million from nongovernmental sources such as foundations, voluntary organizations, and the pharmaceutical industry. About £4 (US$9) per capita is spent each year on medical research.

Having served on several governmental and private grant-giving committees I do not regard these sums as adequate. It is true that very good proposals can usually be funded, but I think it is dangerous to assert that very good proposals are never refused, because the best are likely to come from established research teams that not only excel in research, but in writing plausible applications. There is a danger that the bright young research worker with little or no experience in the art of writing proposals, and with few past achievements to be cited, may not get the support needed to continue in a research career.

Unfortunately, available statistics do not give a breakdown of the proportion of the total funds allocated for pediatric research. It is my impression, however, that the sum is relatively small, partly because the tradition of pediatric research is fairly recent and the number of applications of high quality still limited; partly because the memberships of some of the grant-giving committees do not include individuals with experience in pediatric research and awareness of the ethical constraints peculiar to research on the fetus, the infant, and the older child.

In general, research on the basic aspects underlying child health is better supported than clinical research, but much of this basic research is conducted in one of the institutes or units of the MRC. Fortunately there are some voluntary organizations with a special interest in pediatric research—in particular the National Fund for Research into Crippling Diseases, the Spastics Society, and the Liverpool Children's Research

Fund—and pediatric research is greatly indebted to them. The National Fund has endowed several chairs in pediatrics and has provided funds to establish laboratories for pediatric research.

PEDIATRICS IN THE COMMUNITY

Academics have a special concern for the quality of child health services, not only in the hospital, but in the community. They are particularly concerned about improving the quality of primary care for children, and the need for such improvement is especially great in some of our large cities. In Britain primary care for children is provided by general practitioners rather than by pediatricians. But many academic units now have on their staffs a person with a special interest in the problems of pediatrics in the community, such as school medicine, and in the care of children with physical or mental handicap. It is hoped that these new appointments will help to integrate the three parts of our child health services—primary care, service in the schools and child health clinics, and hospital services. Professor S. Donald M. Court was chairman of a royal commission whose aim was to make recommendations for the improvement of child health services; its report, *Fit for the Future,* appeared in 1976.[2] Unfortunately, not all of its recommendations relating to primary care are likely to be implemented.

Before leaving the subject of child health services in the community, I should say that with one exception the United Kingdom does not have any institutions comparable to your schools of public health. The exception is the London School of Hygiene and Tropical Medicine, one of the units of the University of London. The school is concerned primarily with teaching postgraduates rather than undergraduates.

Most medical schools now have a department of social medicine that has as its function teaching and research in community health, but it does not usually carry responsibility for providing services. In general, however, there is good cooperation between that department and the department of child health in connection with the provision of health services for children in the community.

UNDERGRADUATE TRAINING IN PEDIATRICS[3]

Pediatrics is now regarded by most universities, with the possible exception of London, as one of the five principal clinical subjects, together with medicine, surgery, obstetrics and gynecology, and psychiatry. The student spends from eight to twelve weeks in pediatrics, depending on the medical school. The General Medical Council allows, indeed encourages, experiments with different curricula, so it is therefore not possible to describe a uniform pattern.

In broad outline the curriculum is divided into four parts—premedical, preclinical, clinical, and the preregistration year.

The premedical subjects are usually taken while the students are still in "high school,"* and most universities require competency in three of the four subjects of biology, physics, chemistry, and mathematics. There is a welcome recent trend to allow inclusion of a nonscientific subject.

The preclinical course usually lasts two years and includes anatomy, physiology, the behavioral sciences, genetics, reproduction, and statistics; there is a variable amount of integration with the clinical subjects. Pediatricians usually take part in teaching during this part of the medical course and have the opportunity to emphasize the aspects of the basic sciences that are particularly relevant to child health and pediatrics.

In many medical schools the students are encouraged to spend an intercalated year, following the preclinical course and before starting the clinical course, during which they study certain aspects of one of the basic sciences in greater depth and may have the opportunity to carry out research. A degree of bachelor of science (B.Sc.) may be awarded at the end of that year.

The clinical course usually takes three years, and the main body of instruction in pediatrics and child health takes place during this period. In the final clinical year the student tends to be given increasing clinical responsibility and may be encour-

---

* The United Kingdom has no equivalent of the "college" in the United States. Subjects taken in an American college are covered during the last two years of high school in Britain.

aged to spend an elective period, preferably abroad in a developed or developing country. Instruction takes place not only in the teaching hospital, but often in neighboring nonteaching hospitals and in the community, where it includes an attachment to a general practice. In about half the medical schools pediatric teaching is based in children's hospitals. Instruction consists mainly of bedside and outpatient teaching and seminars for small groups of five to eight students; the formal lecture is being used less than in the past.

After completing the clinical course, and having passed the qualifying examination of which pediatrics is a part, students have to work for one year as preregistration house officers before they are registered. They may then continue with vocational training for whatever branch of medicine they intend to pursue as a career—including general practice.

In only a few medical schools can pediatrics be taken as one of the subjects of the preregistration year, which is usually spent in adult medicine and surgery. Most pediatricians believe that their specialty can provide an excellent educational experience for the preregistration year, provided adequate supervision is available on a twenty-four-hour basis, and that during this period some of the best students may become attracted to pediatrics as a career. During this year, which is regarded as a most important educational experience, students carry full clinical responsibilities. There is, however, some dissatisfaction about the quality and the quantity of the educational experience, particularly because clinical duties tend to be too heavy. In future, academic departments may be given greater responsibility for the supervision of the educational aspects of the preregistration year.

CONCLUSIONS

I hope this has been a satisfactory bird's-eye view of the status of academic pediatrics in the United Kingdom, and that it has touched on some topics of interest. I intentionally highlighted problems we encounter instead of dwelling on successes.

Our chief aim must be to make academic pediatrics an

exciting prospect for some of the best of our medical under-graduates and postgraduates. In order to achieve this we must strive to:

- Enlarge the staffs of the academic departments so there is enough time for research, teaching, and clinical excellence.
- Make more funds available for research fellowships for young investigators.
- Ensure that pediatricians-in-training are not so fully oc-cupied with clinical duties that they have no time for research.
- Prevent our training schedules for pediatricians from becoming too rigid, thereby discouraging them from setting aside a period for research or from traveling to observe and to contribute to practice or research in other parts of the world.
- Ensure that the salary differential of academics and con-sultants does not become too great.
- Lighten the administrative and committee burdens of senior academics, because to many of our younger colleagues the life we lead does not look too attractive.

NOTES

1. S. D. M. Court and A. Jackson, eds. *Paediatrics in the Seventies* (London, New York, Toronto: Published for the Nuffield Provincial Hospitals Trust by the Oxford University Press, 1972): 15.

2. *Fit for the Future*, Report of the Committee on the Child Health Services, S. D. M. Court, chairman (London: Her Majesty's Stationery Office, 1976).

3. *Basic Medical Education in the British Isles*, Report of the General Medical Council Survey of Basic Medical Education in the United Kingdom and Republic of Ireland, 1975–76, 2 vols. (London: Nuffield Provincial Hospitals Trust, 1977): vol. 2, 487–516.

ACADEMIC PEDIATRICS
IN SWITZERLAND AND FRANCE

Ettore Rossi

SWITZERLAND

Switzerland, with a population of 6.5 million, has 700 pediatricians. Half are academicians who teach and staff the hospitals; half are in private practice. Thus, if one considers practicing pediatricians only, the ratio to the population is 1:18,570.

The Swiss medical schools are faculties of the state (cantonal) universities. The medical degree is a federal license, however, which gives the physician the right to practice anywhere in the country. There are five full medical faculties at Basle, Berne, Geneva, Lausanne, and Zurich; one preclinical faculty at Fribourg; and one premedical faculty at Neuchatel.

Undergraduate Education

The total duration of undergraduate medical education is six years, the last being an elective year.

The six-year program is divided into five blocks, followed by national examinations (Table 1). The preclinical period of two years is characterized by an interchange between the two phases of education—natural sciences and human biology, including medical psychology. In the elective year, which in some faculties is the fifth rather than the sixth, a choice of educational programs is offered. They may be taken in clinical or

TABLE 1. DURATION OF UNDERGRADUATE EDUCATION, SWITZERLAND

Year	
1	Natural science
2	Human biology
3	Clinical basic sciences Introduction to clinical subjects
4 5	Clinical clerkships (48 weeks each)
6	Final elective (10 months)

theoretical departments; peripheral hospitals; social service institutions; offices of practicing physicians; or in foreign institutions—there is no limit on location. Horizontal and vertical integration is encouraged: increasingly, clinical and psychosocial subjects are introduced early in the curriculum.

Education in Pediatrics

Pediatric education begins in the third year of the curriculum in the form of introductory clinical tutorials at the bedside, so-called *Gruppenunterricht,* which are characterized by personal contacts with patients. They are conducted by the same tutor, and there are only four or five students in each group. This propaedeutical bedside education takes place one morning a week for five weeks. The student learns to interact with and interview patients and their relatives and to do simple diagnostic bedside procedures.

In the fourth and fifth years, after an introductory course students start the clinical clerkship consisting of 213 hours of lectures. Pediatrics is covered in thirty-two hours over a nine-week period; this will probably be extended. In addition, every week from January to August there are two hours of clinical case presentations in pediatrics, as compared to four hours in internal medicine.

The students then spend six weeks in a pediatrics clerkship: compared to nine weeks in internal medicine, and six each in surgery and gynecology. During the clerkship each student remains in close contact with a patient from admission to discharge. She/he also conducts interviews and performs physical examinations under the supervision of a tutor.

In the final elective year about 25 percent of the students choose pediatrics for a month or more of training.

Postgraduate Education

Postgraduate education in pediatrics lasts for five years. The first year may be taken as a residency in another discipline. The following four consist of a residency in a pediatrics department at a university hospital or in a large peripheral pediatric department. Doctors who are trained in a university department must complete their last year in a peripheral pediatrics department and vice versa.

The pediatrician's academic career begins when the graduate is awarded the degree of *privatdozent* (assistant professor), at which time the council of the medical faculty evaluates the candidate's scientific abilities. After a certain period of continuous scientific activity she/he may be appointed *nebenamtlicher* (part-time professor), but without faculty membership; the next grade is *vollamtlicher* (full professor) with admission to the faculty; and finally, *ordentlicher* (faculty member).

Although the danger of superspecialization clearly exists in Switzerland, making it difficult to select pediatricians as chairmen of university departments, the current prospect for academic pediatrics is good.

A great many pediatricians on every university faculty carry out clinical duties and conduct research on different aspects of the discipline. Clinical activity is supported by the canton; most research is supported by the National Research Foundation, but some funds come from private industry. Pediatric research in fields such as behavioral development, perinatology, and nutrition is completely integrated in these programs. Good contact is also maintained with schools of public health.

With some exceptions, most pediatricians develop clinical investigation programs and are also active members of the clinical staffs of the hospitals.

FRANCE

With a population of approximately 53 million, France has some 2,600 pediatricians, representing a ratio of about 1 per 20,000 population. Sixty percent of the children are seen by general practitioners, however, who are trained in preventive pediatrics and the treatment of prevalent diseases. It is estimated that France will have 3,600 pediatricians by 1990.

Undergraduate Training

Undergraduate education in pediatrics begins in the third and fourth years of medical school with six weeks of bedside tutorials—four hours, three times a week. The training is supervised by a chief medical resident.

During this period practical training is given in vaccinations, cutaneous responses, practical dietetics, nursing assistance, and elementary psychomotor tests. The student is also instructed in the correct physician's response to the parents of sick children. An examination is given at the end of the fourth year.

In the fifth year the student is introduced to practical work on pediatric wards—the internship period. In addition, there are sixty hours of lectures followed by a written examination. The student also attends clinical demonstrations and seminars on diagnostic and therapeutic methods for a period of four to six months, depending on local conditions. In the seventh year a full-time internship in pediatrics is taken by about 10 to 15 percent of students.

Postgraduate Training

Postgraduate education in pediatrics in France is divided into two categories:

• Physicians who have completed a four-year pediatric internship in university hospitals (the equivalent of a residency in the United States) are board-qualified in pediatrics without an additional examination.

• Physicians who do not take a pediatric internship have to take four years of full-time practical courses in pediatrics. They must pass an examination at the end of the first year (*examen régional*), and a final examination at the end of the fourth year (*examen national*).

Beginning in 1983 a new procedure will unite these two systems in France so that a physician who wishes to be certified as a pediatrician will have to:

• Complete a four-year postgraduate internship.

• Attend theoretical and practical courses and pass a national examination.

• Participate in a specific number of national seminars and colloquia.

• Prepare a scientific thesis on a pediatric topic.

Access to an academic career in France requires the following steps:

1. A national jury meets once a year and places a candidate's name on a "national list of competence" as a *Maître de conference* if she/he has successfully passed examinations and hearings and has given satisfactory evidence of scientific work performed.

2. The council of a medical faculty selects one of the pediatricians from the competence list.

3. Finally, the candidate is given the title of titular professor-medical director by the *Comité Consultatif des Universités* (CCU), a national institution with a special Section on Pediatrics and Medical Genetics. Members of the CCU are nominated by the Ministries of Health and Universities.

CONCLUSION

As is apparent, there are pronounced differences between the training processes in Switzerland and France. In fact in both countries many aspects are still in a state of evolution. For example, the procedures for the final examinations in Switzerland, which are at this time being discussed, are still a long way from a satisfactory resolution. The concept of a comprehensive examination may be the solution for the future.

THE FUTURE OF ACADEMIC PEDIATRICS

THE FUTURE OF ACADEMIC PEDIATRICS: WHAT ARE THE NEEDS?

Anne A. Gershon

All is not well in the household of academic medicine in the United States. Recently there has been an alarming decline in the number of medical students and house officers, even those graduating from prestigious medical programs, who are electing academic careers.[1]

This decline may be causally related to at least two phenomena. Perhaps most significant, although intangible, is the perception that society now values science and the scientific method less than it did not long ago. In the first and early second half of the twentieth century it seemed that science could provide the answers to many of society's problems, but large segments of the population have come to view science as part of the problem, rather than the answer; the public has become disillusioned with science. Napalm, Agent Orange, the Love Canal, Three Mile Island, and an acid rain have had a cumulative toxicity on the appeal of science. Faith turns elsewhere. Witness the rise, for example, of astrology in modern America, and the political clout of Laetrile.

Disenchantment with science is linked to the misuse of technology by a callous industrial complex that has grown accustomed to viewing the earth, the air, the rivers, and the oceans as vast cloacas. Every time a chemical dump explodes in New Jersey or a chromosome breakage occurs in Niagara Falls the prestige of science is lessened.

The advanced weaponry used to wreak havoc in an unpopular war linked science not just to war, but to an unwanted war. The military use of science has come to symbolize science for many who forget the development of antibiotics and modern vaccines, but selectively remember the cost in dollars and land devastation of the MX missile program.

To some, science appears malignant, growing out of control. While medicine has remained on the sidelines, it too, has been the victim of an antiscientific backlash resulting in the feeling that the "technology of medicine has outrun its sociology."[2]

Science has been brought under control in medical school curricula. It is controlled so well in fact that little often remains of the basic science years. The lack of laboratory experience that Abraham Flexner complained of in curricula prior to 1910 is almost as much a characteristic of modern medical education as it was then. Consequently we have a new generation of potential and newly educated physicians who have little laboratory experience as the result of "core curricula," and who feel they can achieve status in the eyes of society only by providing health care, preferably through family practice. These medical students may be trained in schools where superb research is conducted, but they exit from their training scientifically deprived and with little inclination to do research themselves.

Even academic clinical faculties contribute to the malaise. Health care services rather than research is pushed as the new wave. In pediatrics we see this expressed by the fact that "ambulatory care" has become a newly discovered "academic discipline." No one can argue about the importance of providing health care, but at some point it is no longer research. In fact in many institutions it is not even academic; it is pure clinical service.

The second reason for the decreasing interest in academic medicine is the availability of funds: money is not now flowing toward academia. Medical students and young investigators cannot help but be aware of the erratic and often inadequate governmental support of academic centers and of research and training. In addition, while once the young investigator could expect to take home a larger salary as a National Institutes of

Health (NIH) fellow than as a resident, this is no longer the case. The ever-widening gap between the remuneration available in private or group practice and that in an academic career, coupled with the increasing high cost of medical education, also do their part to lure young people away from academic medicine—at one major medical school in the Northeast the average 1979 graduate was $20-30,000 in debt. Society seems to be putting its money where its mouth is. It rewards the provision of health care to the rich; thus the bulk of our graduates can be found practicing medicine in affluent locations.

Unfortunately, pediatrics has additional unique difficulties that combine with the general loss of academic attractiveness and create further loss of potential academic pediatricians. Pediatrics is especially affected by the decline in population growth, which has resulted in the birth of fewer children. Moreover its great success in preventive care has brought about decreased utilization of pediatric beds, and this has led to the financial distress of pediatric services.

Finally, there is poorer compensation for pediatrics than its adult counterpart, medicine. There are no Medicare funds available in pediatrics; there is an unwillingness on the part of the public to pay as much for medical care for children as for adults, and pediatricians therefore usually earn less than other medical specialists.

Medical administrators, with eyes fixed on the bottom lines of their budgets, may be tempted to do away with departments of pediatrics. Medical schools should not be run for profit, however, but to serve the needs of society. Children continue to need medical care, and it is clear that the world needs pediatricians and will continue to need them. As stated so well by C. H. Kempe, "children are our future and therefore our most valuable asset."[3]

Pediatric services for sick and well children require as much specialization and talent and as many facilities as adult care units. Academic pediatricians are necessary to provide future training; diagnostic tools; treatments; medical advances for child health; and standards of medical excellence. The decline in academic pediatrics as a career choice is therefore likely to be at least as challenging to future generations as the toxic waste dumped into the Love Canal.

What is to be done? First of course one has to recognize the problem. It seems such a short time ago that research was king and a life of teaching and investigation seemed exciting. To most senior academicians it still is; nothing has changed. They must realize that the world of the children is not the world of the fathers and mothers. We must, after recognizing the unpopularity of our specialty, seek ways to increase its appeal. Academic medicine in general, and pediatrics in particular, should be made more attractive, but these goals cannot be achieved by pediatricians alone.

In order to encourage an interest in academics it is essential to emphasize science, research, and the importance of discovery, as was once done early in the medical school curriculum. Laboratory experience ought to be reinstated in the first two years of medical school. The laboratory not only introduces the student to the scientific method, it provides personal contact with the scientist who teaches there.

Next, we pediatricians must work with governmental agencies to *stabilize* and expand the funding of medical education, research, and training so that secure planning for the future may again become possible.

We must seek ways to improve the financial status of academic pediatricians so they are not forced to give up research and to augment their incomes through private practice.

In order to improve the field, both in terms of service provided and financial betterment, regionalization of pediatric care must be implemented. Sick children should be cared for in medical centers. This approach would deal with the low average utilization of pediatric beds while permitting many advanced services to be maintained. Every hospital does not need a pediatric inpatient service. Regional pediatric centers ought to be located in medical schools and in hospitals that have obstetrical and surgical centers. Obstetrical services should be confined to these centers. High quality pediatric care available in medical centers should have financial parity with high quality medical care provided in the same institutions.

To accomplish this it will be necessary for pediatricians to work with and try to influence third-party payers. Pediatricians should start a campaign to increase public awareness of the importance and successes of pediatric care. The value of preventive medicine and its relationship to science must be emphasized. The public needs to be made aware that scientific medicine has been and is valuable. The dollars, the lives saved, and the misery prevented by such advances as vaccines for poliomyelitis, measles, and rubella, for example, should be stressed so that science is not always linked with expensive equipment.

Finally, it must be recognized that the problems faced by academic pediatrics are not restricted to pediatricians. All of us in academic medicine are involved. No discipline is an island; each is part of the whole. Help must therefore be obtained from medical schools and other branches of medicine. Public policy is involved and must be influenced, and this cannot be done unless we all agree and work together. If the people want good care for their children and their children's children they should be willing to work to change policy in order to provide it.

NOTES

1. J. B. Wyngaarden, "The Clinical Investigator as an Endangered Species," *New England Journal of Medicine* 301 (1979): 1254–59.

2. Ibid.: 1258.

3. C. H. Kempe, "Approaches to Preventing Child Abuse," *American Journal of Diseases of Children* 130 (1976): 941–47.

THE FUTURE OF ACADEMIC PEDIATRICS: WHAT ARE THE RESEARCH NEEDS?

John D. Johnson

I will focus on needs in the area of pediatric research. My first thesis is that to ensure continued advances in research we need to develop means to improve the *recruitment* of pediatrician-investigators, to *train* them, and to sustain and retain them.

There are implications that we are in serious trouble in terms of recruitment. The interest of medical students in research as a career is flagging. At the peak of what D. H. Funkenstein called the "scientific era of medicine," 1959–68, over 45 percent of Harvard medical students assigned a high priority to research; by 1976, the era of primary care and increasing governmental control, only *2 percent* felt research was highly important.[1] A survey by the Association of American Medical Colleges (AAMC) of 7,800 medical students graduating in 1978 revealed that less than 10 percent planned to pursue research fellowship training.[2] The number of physicians in research training programs supported by the National Institutes of Health (NIH) fell from over 4,000 in 1969 to about 1,800 in 1977, and only about 900 new trainees entered the pool in that year.[3] Estimates of the need for physician-investigators as faculty members differ considerably depending on varying basic assumptions; they range from about 800 to over 3,000 a year to replace clinical faculty; a middle estimate by two different types of analysis puts the figure at 1,800.[4] Thus at the present time the training of physician-investigators is barely meeting the *lowest* estimate of perceived needs.

How do these figures apply to academic pediatrics? Over 200 job listings in academic pediatrics appeared in the April 1979 and 1980 issues of *Clinical Research,* and I doubt this list is complete. (I also do not know how critical it is to fill all the listed positions.) The proportion of pediatricians entering academic medicine decreased from 26 percent of those completing their residencies in 1961–64 to 13 percent in 1975–77.[5] If 10 percent of medical students enter the field, and only 10 percent of those go into academic pediatrics, the supply of academic pediatricians will total about 150 a year over the next decade—not enough to fill the faculty positions currently available.

Another way to look at the situation is to apply the same type of analysis the AAMC utilized to assess the need for total clinical faculty. (Table 1)[6] If we assume that there are about 3,500 faculty members in academic pediatrics at the present time (there were 3,266 in 1976–77), that no growth in faculty is needed, that the average length of their active tenure is thirty-five years, and that there is no attrition, then we need 100 new postdoctoral trainees a year; with a 1 percent annual attrition of faculty, the total would be 135 a year; with a 1 percent attrition, and assuming only 75 percent of the trainees become faculty members, the number needed would be 180 a year. About 100 new postdoctoral trainees are currently being supported by the National Institute of Child Health and Human Development (NICHD), many of whom will not become pediatric faculty members. Thus federal support to train academic pediatricians is marginal at best.

TABLE 1. ESTIMATE OF THE NEED FOR
TRAINEES IN ACADEMIC PEDIATRICS

Assumptions	Number of New Trainees Each Year
3,500 faculty members with 35-year tenure, no growth and no attrition.	100
1 percent attrition a year	135
1 percent attrition, plus 75 percent of trainees entering academic pediatrics	180

The declining interest of medical students in research and its reflection in the decreasing number of postdoctoral research trainees probably have multiple origins. Among those often cited are a lack of emphasis on research technique in the medical school undergraduate years; societal pressures favoring careers in primary care—the Manpower Act of 1976, for example; low fellowship stipends, along with their payback provision; and the perception of an unstable career in academic medicine because of growing competition for limited research funds.

There are many possible points of attack to try to reverse these trends. I will allude to a few, and hope that Henry Barnett and William Anlyan will explore them further.

Support for medical student research programs could be expanded. In teaching medical students more emphasis should be placed on research principles and on the fundamental research basis for many clinical observations and diseases. I question the wisdom of the new three-year residency requirement in general pediatrics for the committed pediatrician-investigator.

Fellowship stipends should be increased and the payback provision eliminated—and we should seek training funds from private sources. To ensure a source of highly trained individuals who are prepared for long and productive investigative careers, fellowship programs must be designed to provide rigorous research training, and not be used merely to help meet existing clinical care demands—a trend that has developed to some degree in my own subspecialty of neonatology. Training in biostatistics, experimental design, and the basic sciences related to the clinical research project is essential in the preparation of successful clinical investigators.

Similarly, recruitment at the junior faculty level should not be based solely on meeting patient care loads. Junior faculty need to be nurtured and protected. Sources for research funding at this level could be expanded by, for example, increased funding of the Biomedical Research Support Grant Program and Young Investigators Awards, as well as by foundation support.

In addition to expressing the need for continued input of qualified pediatric researchers, we should ask the question:

Researchers for what kind of research? Is it to be fundamental, untargeted research, unfettered by public desires to address specific health problems? Or is it to be directed by congressional "disease-of-the-month" enthusiasts? Are we capable of defining long-range research priorities, in our case, with regard to child health? The Department of Health and Human Services (DHHS) has adopted a set of health research principles, and the NIH and each of its institutes are developing five-year plans to address research priorities and the allocation of funds according these to priorities.

Many people are skeptical about comprehensive national planning for research. Biologist David Baltimore has stated: "I conclude that society can choose to have either more science or less science, but choosing what science to have is not a feasible alternative."[7] He goes on to say that attempts to control the direction of basic research will result in disruption and demoralization, and that creative people will shun those areas of science in which they know their creativity will be channeled and limited.

In a recent editorial Thomas J. Kennedy, Jr. of the AAMC states that:

> The prevalent impulse to impose "order" and "direction" on an enterprise that depends heavily on the creativity of free spirits and that has been so successful is frightening. . . . I believe that a persuasive case has not been made that proposed extensive changes in existing efforts to plan for biomedical research are worth the cost—in dollars, in time and effort of scientists, and in the risk of further restraining scientific inquiry.[8]

No one would deny that many clinical advances have resulted from apparently unrelated fundamental research, as has been so clearly illustrated by J. H. Comroe, Jr., and R. D. Dripps.[9] Yet in the current era of public accountability and fiscal austerity it seems we have little choice but to accept long-range planning and make the best of it. If long-range planning results in predictability and continuity of research funding it may facilitate the recruitment of talented young investigators to academic pediatrics.

I do not feel that we as pediatricians can justifiably take the same position as Baltimore. In entering pediatrics we make a commitment to the health care priorities of current and future generations of children; thus our research priorities must be guided to some degree by these needs, for, historically, pediatrics has been responsive to societal needs. As the five-year research plan for the NICHD develops, it is to be hoped that broad areas of interest will be defined—almost certainly including those discussed in this conference—and that *within* each of these areas a strong emphasis will be placed on basic exploratory research in developmental phenomena. As the planning of the DHHS proceeds, one trusts that those responsible will realize that such plans should be broad-based, flexible, and responsive to social and scientific changes; that in setting priorities they must take into account not *only* the magnitude of a given health problem, but current scientific knowledge in that area, and thus the opportunity to help solve that health problem; and that the plans should allow for real growth because of the increasing scope of health-related research—they should not be used as a means to place a ceiling on the federal research budget.

In summary, while the kind of research needed in academic pediatrics should be based on child health needs, within broadly defined areas the discovery of knowledge through basic research in developmental biology must be given appropriate emphasis, along with applied clinical research. My hope is that the implementation of research priorities in child health would be mainly through investigator-initiated grants in the priority areas, rather than strictly by the contract mechanism.

NOTES

1. D. H. Funkenstein, *Medical Students, Medical Schools and Society During Five Eras: Factors Affecting the Career Choices of Physicians, 1958–1976* (Cambridge, Massachusetts: Ballinger Publishing Co., 1978).

2. *1978 Medical Student Graduation Questionnaire Survey* (Washington: Association of American Medical Colleges, 1978).

3. J. B. Wyngaarden, "The Clinical Investigator as an Endangered Species," *New England Journal of Medicine* 301 (1979): 1254–59.

4. *Clinical Research Manpower, Report of the Ad Hoc Committee on Clinical Research Training* (Washington: Association of American Medical Colleges, 1980).

5. *The Future of Pediatric Education, Report of the Task Force on Pediatric Education* (Evanston, Illinois: Task Force on Pediatric Education, nd [1978?]).

6. *Clinical Research Manpower* (See note 4).

7. D. Baltimore, "Limiting Science: A Biologist's Perspective," *Daedalus* (Spring 1978): 37–45.

8. T. J. Kennedy, Jr., "Is Comprehensive National Planning for Research Feasible?", *Clinical Research* 28 (1980): 81–84.

9. J. H. Comroe, Jr., and R. D. Dripps, "Scientific Basis for the Support of Biomedical Science," *Science* 192 (1976): 105–09.

THE FUTURE OF ACADEMIC PEDIATRICS: PRIMARY CARE AND COMMUNITY INTERVENTION

David Satcher

There are obviously some differences in definitions relating to academic pediatrics, and therefore I feel it first necessary to define what I mean by the term. Academic pediatrics is that area of pediatrics concerned with improving the health and the health care of children through research, through education, and through exemplary patient care. By the same token I define research as "a systematic approach to the answering of questions or solving of problems"; in this case that would relate to problems and questions dealing with the health and health care of children. I feel that the kind of research needed in pediatrics should not be limited to biomedical or laboratory research, but should include health services and nonbiomedical research; this therefore requires an affiliation of pediatricians and nonbiological scientists, including sociologists, psychologists, and human behaviorists.

My own bias as it relates to the future needs of academic pediatrics has its roots in my personal background and my training in the discipline. I was born and reared in Anniston, Alabama, where my father was a dirt farmer. My mother had nine pregnancies and never saw an obstetrician/gynecologist: all of her babies were delivered by a midwife with no formal training. She had learned midwifery from her mother, who in turn had learned it from her own mother, and so on back through the generations. As a child I became severely ill with whooping cough, which led to pneumonia, and the general practitioner who saw me predicted I would die. But no member of my family ever saw a pediatrician; in fact I never met one until I went to medical school.

My difficulty with academic medicine, and therefore with academic pediatrics, is that at times I have been unable to see the relevance of these disciplines to the unmet needs of children. Therefore I believe the future role of academic pediatrics includes the obligation to respond to the needs of medically underserved children, whether at the biomedical research level or the primary care level. Thus I will limit my comments to the aspects of pediatrics that fall in the area of primary care and community intervention.

The parameters of primary care, as defined by the Committee on Manpower Policy for Primary Health Care of the Institute of Medicine,[1] include accessibility, comprehensiveness, continuity, coordination, and accountability. Now *accessibility* refers to care that is readily available, attainable, and acceptable to the population in question. While we have made great progress in terms of accessibility in the last ten to twenty years, there are areas where care is still not available. In pediatrics this applies especially to the handicapped, to the chronically ill, to adolescents, to the poor, and to minorities. If pediatrics is to be relevant to the needs of underserved communities it must extend itself effectively beyond the boundaries of the academic medical centers.

National Health Service Corps physicians who participated in the Continuing Medical Education Program of Region IV,* for which I have served as a consultant, have described how very ill-prepared they feel when they are sent to provide care to a community that has never had a medical service. In fact graduates from our training programs in academic medical centers are often totally unprepared to function outside that environment. In this sense academic pediatrics and academic medicine are not fulfilling their responsibilities. In order to be

---

* Region IV, so designated by the Department of Health and Human Services, consists of eight states in the Southeast United States.

accessible, pediatrics must begin to go where children live, work, and play, including the home, the school, and athletic programs—as well as the juvenile delinquency system—where the effects of extreme exertion on physical and emotional development remain unanswered questions. All these areas have serious research, training, and service needs.

Comprehensive care generally includes preventive or health promotion activities, diagnosis—especially early diagnosis— treatment, and rehabilitation. Perhaps in no other field of medicine is the need for more emphasis on preventive medicine and health promotion more obvious than in pediatrics, where the early habits and lifestyles of children require supervision and revision. Many chronic illnesses, including hypertension, obesity, and even alcoholism, often have their beginnings in adolescence, and yet it is this age group that tends to be the most neglected. The early diagnosis of many chronic illnesses could conceivably alter their course significantly. Early treatment of addiction, obesity, and hypertension could improve the prognosis for these young people. As a result of our success in genetic diagnosis and early treatment, a growing population of children are requiring special rehabilitation and treatment services, and it remains for academic pediatrics to begin to solve the problems that relate to providing them.

Perhaps no parameter of primary care is in greater need of serious consideration and improvement by academic pediatrics than *continuity of care*. Experience with continuity of care during the training of pediatric residents and medical students is critical for a comprehension of human growth and development. Not only is it difficult to understand human growth and development without extended contact with patients of different ages and at different stages of development, but in terms of research one cannot ask the right questions or begin to solve the problems without experience in continuity of care. A needs assessment study conducted in the Watts section of Los Angeles in 1975 clearly demonstrated that one matter of most concern to consumers is a continuing relationship with providers in the health care system.[2]

The next parameter of primary care is *coordination*. The pediatrician is certainly not alone in providing care to children;

patients must be guided through a very complicated system in order to receive comprehensive services. The health care team must be used more effectively, not only in patient care, but in research and in education. If the health care team is used to the greatest advantage this will certainly extend the ability of the pediatrician to give comprehensive care.

Persons such as nurse practitioners, physicians' assistants, social workers, and nutritionists certainly can add significantly to the care of children if the pediatrician relates to them appropriately. It is up to academic pediatrics to prepare pediatricians to work effectively with health care teams, and to begin to ask the questions and to solve the problems that now prevent effective utilization of such teams.

In the area of *accountability*, academic pediatrics, like every other field of academic medicine, must begin to look more critically at the outcome of clinical medicine. It is becoming increasingly clear that too little effort has gone into evaluating the impact of services rendered on health status or health behavior. In the future, academic pediatrics must prepare pediatricians to assess the quality of the outcome of care as well as to take advantage of the skills of others doing so.

In short, academic pediatrics must consider the fact that over 75 percent of pediatricians practice general pediatrics;[3] even those involved in subspecialty pediatrics spend most of their time providing general services. In the training of pediatric residents this fact must always be considered in planning the trainees' experiences and developing the objectives of the training program.

Finally, as a family physician I feel it is important to discuss briefly the pediatrics-family practice interface. First it is important to remember that the majority of American children are not cared for by pediatricians; over 50 percent of children who seek medical services receive care from either a general practitioner or a family physician.[4] All the present evidence suggests that in the future the number of family physicians will increase. Academic pediatrics will therefore have a very important role to play in the training of physicians other than pediatricians to care for children.

Later this year, as a representative of the Society of

Teachers of Family Medicine, I will be meeting with committees of the American Academy of Family Practice (AAFP) and the American Academy of Pediatrics (AAP) to discuss the pediatric objectives for family practice residency training; in their approach to this issue the three groups are not too far apart. The AAFP has recommended that a minimum of five months of family practice residency training be spent in pediatrics, and that 18 to 20 percent of the patients seen in family practice model units be in the pediatric age group.

Two years ago the Task Force on Pediatric Education recommended that a minimum of six months of the family practice residents' training be in primary pediatrics under the supervision of the department of pediatrics.[5] The only problem with this recommendation is that many pediatric residents are not given six months' training in primary care pediatrics. We must therefore be skeptical about our ability to provide family practice residents with such an experience. Perhaps this indicates that the training in primary pediatrics of the family practice resident and the pediatric resident will improve simultaneously. In family practice we are dedicated to meeting the health care needs of individuals and families regardless of age or sex; thus our interest in the pediatric age group relates to this basic commitment.

In many of the discussions at this conference it has been implied that family practice is interested only in service. Academic family medicine has in fact its own set of unanswered questions and unsolved problems that relate to the health of individuals and families. We certainly realize the need to collaborate with those in other disciplines, including basic scientists and social, behavioral, and other nonbiological scientists, as we attempt to solve the problems of health and health care delivery to children and to members of their families. Thus it is my hope that more cooperation between family physicians and pediatricians will become evident in the future, and that the growth and progress of academic pediatrics will continue at an accelerated pace.

NOTES

1. Committee on Manpower Policy for Primary Health Care, Institute of Medicine, *Manpower Policy for Primary Health Care* (Washington: National Academy of Sciences, May 1978).

2. D. Satcher, J. Kosecoff, and A. Fink, "Results of a Needs Assessment Strategy in Developing a Family Practice Program in an Inner-City Community," *Journal of Family Practice* 10 (May 1980): 871–79.

3. "Education and the Pediatric Practice System," in *The Future of Pediatric Education, Report of the Task Force on Pediatric Education* (Evanston, Illinois: Task Force on Pediatric Education, nd [1978?]): 38–43.

4. Ibid.: 96–97.

5. Ibid.: 34–35.

DISCUSSANT:

Henry L. Barnett

Professor Philip Morrison of the Massachusetts Institute of Technology, in a commencement address given in 1960 at the Albert Einstein College of Medicine, described in elegant terms some of the developmental processes that took place in the early history of man. The principles underlying his thesis continue to apply, and probably at a progressively increasing rate. Morrison said, for example, that at a time when man's physical world was limited to a small area he had full knowledge of every stone, tree, valley, and hill in that space. As his world expanded so did his resources, and his life was enriched by a great variety of experiences. For this gain, however, he gave up some of the security associated with his familiarity with his former physical world and was faced with new uncertainties that disturbed his previous tranquility.

The term trade-off is used to describe this developmental process, which is actually a form of quid pro quo with a feedback loop. Has it occurred in academic pediatrics? I believe it has, and that we are continuing to undergo such changes. If correct, I would argue that in considering our needs for the future we must recognize the occurrence of such processes in the past. I would suggest also that in the evolution of academic medicine in general over the past sixty years, pediatrics has at several points served as the pioneer among clinical disciplines in broadening the scope of academic concerns and responsibilities.

Many of the most important contributions of biomedical science to clinical medicine during the post-Flexner period, which H. K. Farber and R. McIntosh have called "pediatric biochemistry flowers,"[1] were made by academic investigators in pediatrics. Many people were attracted to the specialty in part because of its preeminence as a scientific clinical discipline. They were relatively comfortable in their familiarity with the nature of the questions that needed answers and with the biomedical tools available with which to investigate them.

A decade or so later, however, many of the problems of acute illnesses were being solved, and those of chronic illnesses and disabilities were becoming more prominent. It was at this time that some leaders in academic pediatrics began to respond to the expressed needs of children and of their families for professional help with new problems, especially those of a psychosocial, behavioral nature. Prominent among these pioneers were Charles A. Aldrich and Milton J. E. Senn, who had begun their academic careers as biomedical clinical investigators. As a result of their influence, and that of others, academic pediatrics was among the early clinical disciplines to extend its concerns to include attempts to understand and treat psychosocial problems of children and their families. In the process, like early man expanding his physical world, academic pediatricians gained new insights and new satisfactions in these more complex fields, but at the same time they forfeited some of the security they had had in the process of treating acute physical illnesses.

A more recent expansion of the scope of academic pediatrics has been the focus on the provision of health services, especially primary care and community intervention. This process also represents a response to expressed changing needs of patients, and academic pediatricians are again playing a prominent innovative role in exploring them. They have accepted the new challenges with enthusiasm. Whether or not they realize it, however, I believe they, too, are giving up some of their former security, and they should have at least some element of uncertainty about their approach to these new tasks.

As a pediatrician who began his academic career in biomedical research forty years ago, I understand what prompted these developments, and as chairman of an academic department of pediatrics, I welcomed and supported programs that broadened its scope, concerns, and responsibilities in patient care, teaching, and research. But in reviewing these events I have two major misgivings that I believe must be taken into account as we consider future needs.

In my judgment we have made two serious errors. First, in expanding our role we have failed to maintain gains of earlier periods. This failure has been most apparent in the decline, if not in the quantity then certainly in the quality, of biomedical and clinical research in academic departments of pediatrics. Despite some disclaimers I believe pediatricians should deplore the contrast between the quality of the scientific programs of their own academic societies and those of internal medicine.

The second error is that too often we have undertaken new roles as amateurs. The pediatrician has a built-in advantage in dealing with psychosocial problems of children and their families, as well as in developing and evaluating the effectiveness of health services, especially in the area of prevention. Too frequently the teaching and practice in these areas has been conducted almost completely intuitively, however, without any attempt to become familiar with or apply the expanding body of knowledge now available, and without seeking collaboration with professionals in related fields such as psychology, sociology, anthropology, and epidemiology.

As a good discussant I have to this point considered neither the subject nor the presentations I have been assigned to discuss. Let me do so in the brief time remaining.

Gershon and Johnson both focused on the future needs of academic pediatrics principally in relation to the research component of academic medicine, and they asked how the present need to recruit and support more investigators can be met. I am both pleased and relieved that Anylan will be answering those questions, and I look forward, as always, to hearing his advice. I would suggest only that the recent increased awareness of the importance of obstetrical and pediatric implications for some adult disorders may stimulate those who determine the use of research funds to be more receptive to requests for support of work related to mothers, to their fetuses, and to infants, children, and adolescents. Adults, including legislators, are interested primarily in diseases that affect them, and they should be made aware that, although they will not die of human development, they could die of some diseases that may originate in early life.

According to Satcher, the role of academic pediatrics, today and tomorrow, is to prepare pediatricians and other physicians to meet the health care needs of children, with special emphasis on those needs that are clearly unmet and underserved. I agree with him that preparing pediatricians and other physicians for the primary care of children and for community intervention is a major responsibility of academic pediatrics. I am certain, however, he would agree that we also have a responsibility to develop new knowledge through research and to train future investigators.

Satcher's presentation raises the question of the relationship between primary and tertiary pediatric care. In my opinion these two types of care are becoming so divergent, in their content, in their educational and training requirements for gaining competence, and in their sources of satisfaction for the respective practitioners, that they are becoming almost separate disciplines. I am not equating primary care with ambulatory care, since it should include care of hospitalized patients either by the primary care physician alone or in consultation with tertiary care pediatricians. Moreover I am not defining tertiary care pediatricians solely as system specialists, since there are, and probably will continue to be, tertiary care generalists.

I do believe, however, that true tertiary care will be given increasingly by organ system specialists appropriately trained to provide consultative care for the increasingly complex chronic diseases of children, and to do both laboratory and clinical research on their pathogenesis, etiology, and prevention. This trade-off, which redefines both the content and the practitioners of primary and tertiary pediatric care, involves even more complex changes than the earlier ones. Whether we like it or not, however, until it is accepted as a necessary developmental change, I do not believe we can define properly the future needs of academic pediatrics.

In summary, I have argued that, since it became separated from internal medicine, academic pediatrics has undergone successive changes in filling important unmet needs. In doing so it has suffered losses, but it has also gained strengths, some of which are yet to be solidified. Its future needs require more precise and realistic definitions of the content of primary and tertiary pediatric care and of the appropriate practitioners; substantial expansion of both the quantity and quality of developmental biomedical research; and greater professionalism in the teaching and training of practitioners and investigators in all areas of pediatrics.

NOTE

1. H. K. Farber and R. McIntosh, *History of the American Pediatric Society, 1887–1965.* (New York: McGraw Hill Book Publishing Co., 1966): *Period 3: 1914–1926,* 93–145.

THE FUTURE OF ACADEMIC PEDIATRICS: HOW DO WE MEET THE NEEDS?

William G. Anlyan

Living everyday in the microcosm of academic pediatrics, surrounded by other clinical specialties that may be more lucrative, it is relatively easy to overlook the positives and become overwhelmed by the negatives. Academic pediatrics in the United States is in a relatively healthy condition; in facing the 1980s it may require certain adjustments rather than a bloody revolution.

THE REALITIES OF THE 1980s

What is the macropicture and the likely scenario for the 1980s within which we have to plan *all* of academic medicine?

• The general economy is in a decade of limited growth, so we have to look for judgmental substitutions rather than a continuing series of add-ons.

• There will be an excess of physicians. The number of slots available in approved residency training programs will come close to the number of physicians graduating.

• In coping with the uncertainties of the nature of medicine in general in the 1990s, there should be no major change in the number of pediatricians produced for primary, secondary, or tertiary subspecialty care. If we were living in the year 1946 our manpower and specialty projections for the late 1950s and 1960s would have included specialists in poliomyelitis and other infectious diseases that are now preventable. Today the key issue to focus on is assurance of the production of adequate numbers of high-quality clinical investigators in pediatrics—more on this later.

• There will be an increase in the "industrialization and collectivization of medicine." Health maintenance organizations (HMOs) and independent practice associations (IPAs) will have a greater impact on the academic medical center and its traditional patient referral patterns. Those centers that stay aloof from HMOs/IPAs will increasingly become tertiary care institutions and will need to expand their educational resources to community hospitals and clinics. Centers that elect to become an integral part of HMOs/IPAs may experience a decrease in referrals from physicians who are not members of the same corporation.

Big business is becoming an active partner in shaping health care policy and options. General Motors and the Ford Motor Company combined spend $1.8 billion a year on health services—close to 1 percent of total American health care expenditures—and they are seeking the best buy with those dollars. Insurance companies heretofore not involved in health are promoting health care packages, including HMOs.

• The marketplace in medicine is beginning to take effect. Medium-sized communities are witnessing the departure of recently arrived physicians who are unable to make an adequate living in these locations. In large multidisciplinary group practices the nonpediatricians are threatening to refer their pediatric patients to another group if fees are not kept at a competitive level.

• The fee-for-service system is being challenged by generalist physicians whose armamentarium does not include special procedures. Instead, a "taximeter" approach is being suggested, similar to that of the legal profession; the meter rate would be adjusted according to such factors as skills, experience, and time expended.

Given the foregoing general trends, what can be done to meet the needs of academic pediatrics in the 1980s and 1990s? First let us look at the existing assets and liabilities.

Existing Assets of Academic Pediatrics

Unlike family practice, pediatrics has a stable and unchallenged place in the mosaic of the academic medical center. It enjoys overlapping areas of mutual concern with all the basic sciences and increasing interdependence with other clinical services. In any given academic medical center the number of pediatric faculty may appear small compared to those in surgery and medicine, but the quality of the faculty is of the highest caliber, comparable to internal medicine in a spectrum that ranges from the clinical investigator to the clinical subspecialist. In general—and possibly by a process of self-selection—academic pediatricians tend to be team players who have little difficulty in collaborative efforts involving departments with which they interface. Statistics of the past decade demonstrate a doubling of pediatric faculty in American medical schools.

Major Liability of Academic Pediatrics

Like family practice, pediatrics in the medical center is the "poor clinical cousin." Income generated from patient care is insufficient to support or backstop other academic activities, including new ventures such as pump-priming young faculty or new programs. Academic pediatrics today cannot be financially self-sufficient without institutional or external funding.

OUTLOOK AND POSSIBLE SOLUTIONS

National

• Federal support for research or research training/fellowships will be distributed among fewer institutions. The institutions that do receive federal support will devote considerable effort to professionalizing research training through such mechanisms as M.D.-Ph.D. programs and academic scholar residency programs. The "dabbler" who savors fundamental research in the postresidency period will fall by the wayside, although there may continue to be some exceptional late bloomers.

My personal view is that the leaders of the National Institutes of Health and its institutes are doing the very best job possible with the monies available. Federal programs for patient care will need to address the inequities of compensation for services rendered by pediatricians and family practitioners vis-à-vis procedure-oriented physicians.

• The private sector has to recognize the special needs of academic pediatrics. The recent trend of a few foundations to provide support to young, promising, potential academicians is to be lauded; these represent very high multiplier programs that will assure the production of future faculty leaders. In contrast to foundations, with a few notable exceptions corporate support has been disappointing. One possible approach to relate to corporations in areas of mutual interest would be to develop "corporate family well-ness" programs. The pediatrician would constitute a key member of the health team treating the total family and observing the potential negative domino effect on the children of the unhappy top corporate executive. Such programs not only offer clinical services and provide opportunities for preventive health education, but are amenable to evaluation and research.

National pediatrics organizations should recognize the flexibility required in special residency training programs for the potential clinical investigator. It is strongly desirable to recruit to such programs residents who began their research experience while in medical school and who are willing to accept a residency program that is longer in duration, but well supported, with a continuing research involvement.

The State and the Local Community

There is no question about the need to increase state and local community resources to support activities championed by academic departments of pediatrics, including patient care programs such as those for crippled children; regionalized health care programs for high-risk pregnancies; research programs for diseases such as cancer and cystic fibrosis; and programs such as health education in schools.

Institutional Responsibility

The department of pediatrics should be regarded by the chief executive officer of the academic medical center as a special entity. Pediatrics deserves a level of institutional support comparable to that given to the basic sciences. Today, unlike other clinical departments, pediatrics cannot "bank" venture funds or make proportionate contributions to capital improvements. In regions where it is legal the teaching hospital can assist by giving partial support to key administrative and supervisory efforts of the pediatric staff.

The future for academic pediatrics need not be "more of the same." In both public and private medical centers, the chief executive officers, departmental chairmen, and key faculty members should engage in substantial fund-raising activities among individuals and institutions in the private sector. Children are our future, and the sick child has a special appeal to the potential benefactor. While the grateful patient may be a minor and the parents young, low-income earners, they are surrounded by grandparents, friends, and neighbors who may be affluent. The greatest asset for our future lies in the private sector and, in particular, in estate planning.

In summary, as responsible academic administrators it is up to us to help create an atmosphere that provides for the optimum continued development of academic pediatrics.

PARTICIPANTS

William G. Anlyan, M.D.
Vice President for Health Affairs
Duke University Medical Center
Durham, North Carolina

Mary Ellen Avery, M.D.
Thomas Morgan Rotch
  Professor of Pediatrics
Harvard Medical School
Children's Hospital Medical Center
Boston, Massachusetts

Henry L. Barnett, M.D.
Professor
Department of Pediatrics
Albert Einstein College of Medicine
  of Yeshiva University
Bronx, New York

Floyd W. Denny, M.D.
Professor and Chairman
Department of Pediatrics
School of Medicine
University of North Carolina
Chapel Hill, North Carolina

Leon Eisenberg, M.D.
Professor and Chairman
Department of Preventive and
  Social Medicine
Harvard Medical School
Boston, Massachusetts

Ilene Fennoy, M.D.
Department of Pediatrics
College of Physicians and Surgeons
Columbia University
Harlem Hospital Center
New York, New York

Anne A. Gershon, M.D.
Associate Professor
Department of Pediatrics
School of Medicine
New York University
New York, New York

Bernard G. Greenberg, M.D.
Dean
School of Public Health
University of North Carolina
Chapel Hill, North Carolina

Melvin M. Grumbach, M.D.
Professor and Chairman
Department of Pediatrics
School of Medicine
University of California,
  San Francisco
San Francisco, California

Robert J. Haggerty, M.D.
President
William T. Grant Foundation
New York, New York

Horace L. Hodes, M.D.
Distinguished Service Professor
Department of Pediatrics
The Mount Sinai Medical Center
New York, New York

John D. Johnson, M.D.
Associate Professor
Department of Pediatrics
School of Medicine
The University of New Mexico
Albuquerque, New Mexico

Jerome Kagan, Ph.D.
Professor of Social Relations
Harvard University
Cambridge, Massachusetts

Edwin L. Kendig, Jr., M.D.
Professor of Pediatrics
Medical College of Virginia
Virginia Commonwealth University
Director
Department of Pediatrics
St. Mary's Hospital
Richmond, Virginia

Norman Kretchmer, M.D., Ph.D.
Director
National Institute of Child Health
   and Human Development
National Institutes of Health
Bethesda, Maryland

John W. Littlefield, M.D.
Given Professor and Chairman
Department of Pediatrics
School of Medicine
The Johns Hopkins University
The Children's Medical and
   Surgical Center
The Johns Hopkins Hospital
Baltimore, Maryland

Dominick P. Purpura, M.D.
Professor and Chairman
Department of Neuroscience
Director
Rose F. Kennedy Center for
   Research in Mental Retardation
   and Human Development
Albert Einstein College of Medicine
   of Yeshiva University
Bronx, New York

Mortimer G. Rosen, M.D.
Professor and Director
Department of Obstetrics and
   Gynecology
Cleveland Metropolitan General
   Hospital

School of Medicine
Case-Western Reserve University
Cleveland, Ohio

Ettori Rossi, M.D.
Professor and Chairman
Department of Pediatrics
Klinik für Kinderkrankheiten
University of Berne
Berne, Switzerland

Joseph W. St. Geme, Jr., M.D.
Professor and Executive Chairman
Department of Pediatrics
School of Medicine
University of California, Los Angeles
Harbor General Hospital Campus
Torrance, California

David Satcher, M.D., Ph.D.
Professor and Chairman
Department of Community Medicine
   and Family Health
School of Medicine
   at Morehouse College
Atlanta, Georgia

Michael A. Simmons, M.D.
Associate Professor
Department of Pediatrics
School of Medicine
The Johns Hopkins University
Baltimore, Maryland

Margaret H.D. Smith, M.D.
Professor of Pediatric Infectious
   Diseases
Department of Pediatrics
School of Medicine
Tulane University
New Orleans, Louisiana

Otto H. Wolff, M.D., F.R.C.P.
Nuffield Professor of Child Health
Institute of Child Health
University of London
London, England

INDEX

Aberrant development, diagnostic procedures for, 106–11

The Abuse of Maternity (Evans), 101

Academia, financial links to government, 23–28

Academic medicine

and availability of funds, 206–07

and disenchantment with science, 205–06

federal support, trends in, 25–26

and National Health Service, United Kingdom, 189–92

and research findings, 26–28

See also Academic pediatrics; Medical schools

Academic pediatrics

assets and liabilities, 228

and Carnegie Commission on Children, recommendations, 45–46

challenges to, 38–42

concerns of department heads, 19

contributions to research, 9–11

in France, 201–02

and levels of patient care, 41

outlook, 228–30

prescription for change, 4–5

proposals for, 208–09

and public health schools, 164–73

and realities of 1980s, 226–28

research expansion, 2–3

research needs, 210–14

residency, 185

role model for students, 56–57

role of private foundations in, 46–48

support of NIH institutes for, 29–33

in Switzerland, 198–200

training, adequacy of, 3–4

and women in medicine, 8–9

See also Medical schools; Obstetrics and gynecology departments; Residency

Accountability, in primary care, 219

Acute illness clinic, and residency, 181

Adolescent medicine, 78–81

Ainsworth, M. D. S., 102

Alcohol, Drug Abuse, and Mental Health Administration, 34

Aldrich, Charles A., 222

Aldrich, Robert A., 4

Ambulatory Pediatric Association, 186

American Academy of Family Practice (AAFP), 220

American Academy of Pediatrics (AAP), 178, 186, 220

American Board of Pediatrics (ABP), 59, 178, 187

American Heart Association, 136

American Journal of Obstetrics and Gynecology, 73

American Medical Association (AMA), 178

American Pediatric Society (APS), 4, 18, 186

Amino acids, and infant nutrition, 133–34

Anlyan, William, 212

Association of American Medical Colleges (AAMC), 23, 25, 26, 30, 210, 211

Association of Pediatric Department Chairmen, 43

233